Gentle Babies

Essential Oils and Natural Remedies for Pregnancy, Childbirth, Infants and Young Children

FOURTH EDITION

Debra Raybern

growing
HEALTHY
HOMES

ISBN: 978-0-9816954-0-2
Printed in the United States of America
Fourth printing.

Growing Health Homes LLC
837 Crown Drive
Bartlesville, OK 74006

To obtain additional copies of this book, please visit
www.GrowingHealthyHomes.com.

Required disclaimer: The information given in this book is for educational purposes only and is not intended as diagnosis, treatment or prescription for any disease. Though essential oils have been used for centuries with only beneficial results and the contributors have all experienced powerful benefits from their usage, the reader is advised to seek the advice of his or her chosen health professional before using essential oils. The content of this book does not necessarily reflect the views of Young Living Essential Oils, LC, Lehi, UT, (YL) and is produced by Independent Distributors. All trademarks are used by permission. The author, publisher, contributors and YL bear no responsibility for the use or misuse of any of these products. The decision to use or not to use any of this information is the sole responsibility of the reader. Also, any and all recommendations for essential oils apply only to YL.

To Sharon and her future blessings.

To Paul – You are greatly missed.

Dedication

For all the moms and moms-to-be around the globe who wish to choose a more natural approach to motherhood and believe being pregnant is not an illness, but rather a joyous time in their lives as they wait for their blessings to arrive.

"Thy wife shall be as a fruitful vine by the sides of thine house; thy children like olive plants round about thy table." Psalm 128:3

Table of Contents

Acknowledgements

Thank you to the many moms who have used therapeutic-grade essential oils with great success and shared those testimonies and suggestions that have made this book possible.

Thank you to D. Gary Young, N.D., for establishing Young Living Essential Oils, so we may share in the goodness of true essential oils. Without these oils this book would never have been written.

Thank you specifically to Beverly Boytim, Karen Douglas and Sera Johnson for recording the essential oils and other natural products as they used them to see what worked and what did not.

Thank you to Hasso Wittboldt-Mueller, N.D., whose handout first inspired me to collect more oil suggestions and write this book.

Thank you Laura Hopkins for her editing and design assistance.

Thank you Growing Healthy Homes LLC for publishing this small, but awesome book.

Thank you to my daughter, Sharon, who sacrificed the most by allowing her mom the time it took to complete this book.

Thank you to my Lord and Savior Jesus Christ, who put me on a path that included this book.

Debra Raybern

Debra Raybern, N.D., M.H., C.N.C., I.C.A.

Important Information

The pure therapeutic-grade essential oils and natural products referenced in this book are exclusively produced by Young Living Essential Oils (YL). After much careful research and study, it is the opinion of the author and contributors that no other brand of essential oil has the power and purity that is an absolute must for everyone, but especially for pregnant and nursing moms and young children.

> *"Wherefore I put thee in remembrance that thou stir up the gift of God, which is in thee by the putting on of my hands. For God hath not given us the spirit of fear; but of power, and of love and of a sound mind." II Timothy 1:6-7*

The Greek word used in this passage for fear is deilia, meaning timidity, and its root deilos, is defined as faithless. This fear is not external, but an internal struggle. According to D. Gary Young, founder of YL, "F-E-A-R is a false emotion appearing real." Use the oils recommended in this book full of faith and without timidity. Thousands of mothers already have.

Foreword

In 1991, I became aware of aromatherapy and essential oils when I was searching for complementary and alternative therapies for my daughter. When my little girl was born she swallowed meconium, the tar-like bowel movement of infants, and it poisoned her system. At seven months old she had a severe case of pneumonia, and she literally died in my husband's arms as we rushed to the hospital. God miraculously gave her back to us. We lived in critical care unit of the hospital for 10 days.

When she was three, a team of doctors told me she was retarded and nothing could be done for her. I refused to accept their diagnosis and started investigating alternatives in health and nutrition. If someone said they had something to help my daughter, I immediately checked it out. One day I got a phone call from a friend, Mary, asking if I knew anything about aromatherapy. She told me about the company Young Living, and its founder Gary Young. She suggested I try two essential oils blends, Peace & Calming and Clarity. When I found research by Dr. Jean-Claude LaPraz examining the effects of essential oils, I was so impressed I began experimenting with Young Living's essential oils with my daughter. My husband and I were overjoyed as we saw significant, positive changes in her abilities. The changes were so substantial, her teachers and the parents of her friends started asking me what I was doing. It was amazing to watch my daughter's progress. She went from being diagnosed as retarded to graduating from college.

The wisdom I gained over the years enabled me to I choose the right information, to grow my mind and take care of my family and myself. This is why I invest thousands of dollars a year on books, tapes and DVDs that provide knowledge.

Gentle Babies is filled with knowledge of the most important nature; it is about you, and how to take care of yourself and your family with essential oils and natural remedies. This wonderful, innovative book by a gifted, generous and intelligent writer will support you and your family with the use of essential oils in your everyday lives. I wholeheartedly recommend it to every family to better their health and as an added resource in their home.

— Marcella Vonn Harting,
Ph.D. candidate in Psychoneurology & Integrative Medicine

•••••

The use of essential oils dates back to ancient times, however there has never been a time when essential oils are more needed in our society than today. The overuse of modern-day 'wonder' drugs has created a potentially hazardous time in our world, more so than the medical science community ever anticipated.

Fortunately, there are answers that provide a way for us to protect ourselves, our family and friends from these potential dangers. The answer is using pure, therapeutic-grade essential oils.

As you can imagine, during our 12 years of using the Young Living products on a daily basis, not only have we gained a better way of life through wellness and longevity, we have enjoyed many incredible experiences. As this book has been dedicated to pregnancy, childbirth and infant care, I would like to share some experiences we have had with our grandchildren and the YL products.

We were at our summer cabin and had one of our daughters and her family with us for the weekend. Their youngest son was just a few months old and was suffering from a high fever. I opened my oil bag and proceeded to administer oils on his little body. I used YL's spearmint oil on his back, stomach, forehead and temples and feet several times within an hour. Then, I soaked a wash cloth in cool water with peppermint added and wiped this cloth over him, cooling his body, careful not to make him chill. I also put spearmint in the bath water and let him soak in the tub until the water was cool, then rubbed R.C. on his chest and feet. This broke his fever, and he was back to normal within a couple of hours.

Our youngest daughter used the YL essential oils and supplements throughout her two pregnancies. She used them for nausea and to prevent stretch marks of which she, a petite redhead, has none after two children. She used the supplements to help keep her body functioning properly while giving good nutrition to her baby. She used them at time of labor with great success. She used them at the time of birth, anointing the babies with frankincense right away and using myrrh on the umbilical cords for protection from infections, as well as to help with the healing. She incorporated the oils Debra mentions in this book, plus others of her choice as she felt inspired to use them.

We have another grandson who from birth had a runny nose and nothing seemed to help. When he was about three years old we gave him a drink of NingXia Red. He liked it and wanted more, and his runny nose stopped and never returned. This was just another confirmation of the power of YL's essential oils and essential-oil-enhanced products.

We became acquainted with Debra many years ago and knew she was someone very special. It has been a delight to see her growth in YL. She has achieved immense success in her search for natural wellness. Her dedication in helping others find natural health and wellness through traditional naturopathic, herbal and essential oils is to be commended.

Well done, Debra. I will consider it a privilege to have your book in my library and will certainly share it with others. I am sure you will see the day when the information contained herein will be mainstay for the masses.

— Shauna Dastrup, friend and associate in the 'Journey of Health, Wellness and Prosperity

• • • • •

Having had the opportunity to study with Daniel Pénoël, M.D., Jean-Claude LaPraz, M.D. and the physicians at the First Aromatic Medicine Congress in Grasse, France, I asked these experts about contraindications during pregnancy. I was assured by each of those I interviewed that essential oils are safe for pregnant women and that essential oils could, in fact, offer many benefits.

I often share this information with students in classes so that if a woman realizes she is pregnant, she will not become overly concerned about the oils she might have used before she found out about her pregnancy. In the fourteen years that I have been using and sharing essential oils, I know many, many women who have used essential oils prolifically during pregnancy with excellent results and no observable detrimental effects.

I understand that we may not know everything about essential oils safety, yet, and I encourage women to use oils responsibly and always err on the side of caution. I suggest that women refrain from purposely using substantial amounts of essential oils during pregnancy and use those oils which have withstood the test of time. Additionally, it may be prudent to consider the contraindication lists that have been created in literature available to us and, whenever possible, adhere to these guidelines.

It is time for us to embrace a healing modality which may have profound benefits for women and their families. Debra Raybern has created a book containing a wealth of information about how women everywhere can safely use essential oils to help themselves and their families live longer, healthier and happier lives. On behalf of women everywhere, I thank you, Debra, for writing this book for us.

— Vicki Opfer, C.N.C.

Introduction

*"And it came to pass that, when Elisabeth heard the greeting
of Mary, the babe leaped in her womb..." Luke 2:41*

Pregnancy is one of the most joyful times in a woman's life. At a time when conventional medicine and therapies often are contraindicated, the use of natural protocols and therapeutic-grade essential oils can assist the soon-to-be-mom with a wide variety of health challenges and experiences such as nausea, stress, labor, delivery and afterbirth care for both mom and baby.

Books on the subject of aromatherapy during pregnancy vary widely in suggestions. One reason for this is the three separate models of aromatherapy: German, British and French. The German model emphasizes inhalation and always extreme dilution. The British model also recommends dilution, but concentrates more on the massage benefits. The French model will use both of these and oral ingestion of therapeutic, grade-A essential oils. The work of Daniel Pénoël, M.D., "Natural Home Health Care Using Essential Oils," 1998, showed taking specific essential oils into the body was not only safe but very effective when other modalities were not.

Essential oil pioneer and globally known expert in the field of growing, harvesting, distilling, blending and usage of essential oils, D. Gary Young has traveled the world learning from each model. As the founder of Young Living Essential Oils (YL), he has combined the best of each model to bring us a unique way of using essential oils plus new, innovative techniques empowering people worldwide to take charge of their health and wellness.

This book suggests combining all modalities, but the safety and effectiveness of these recommendations are found only by using YL's brand of therapeutic-grade essential oils. Because of the purity and quality of these specific oils, the contributors of this book do not endorse any other brand of essential oils.

In the words of Dr. Pénoël, "I'd rather have a single drop of genuine essential oil than a 55 gallon drum of junk product."

All of the recipes and recommendations in this book have been used on thousands of mothers and their babies and children with no ill effects. From time to time a standard herbal suggestion also will be included. These have been selected for their safety and effectiveness.

I applaud you for taking the time to learn more about your family's health and how you can use God's original medicine – essential oils – to have vibrant health. Using natural remedies requires more effort than the conventional thinking of "take this pill and call me in the morning." The time you spend will be well worth your health and that of your family.

I hope you will begin to experience the hundreds upon thousands of daily benefits of using essential oils and essential oils products for health, home and body. This is a very self-empowering process; it is a joy to be able to take responsibility for our own health and see the wonderful benefits. Please jot down your notes and findings as you use these products.

It is likely that this book will be a never-ending project as more families benefit from and share their successes. Please share testimonials with me via editor@growinghealthyhomes.com.

Precautions

Only use essential oils from Young Living Essential Oils (YL), that guarantees to provide only 100 percent pure, therapeutic-grade (YLTG™) oils produced from carefully identified plants with natural chemical profiles that match or exceed recognized world standards. In addition, YL has its own more comprehensive, rigorous internal standard, which is an essential prerequisite to gain therapeutic results without producing harmful side effects.

Avoid citrus oils on skin areas that are exposed to direct sunlight for at least 12 hours to avoid photosensitivities.

Dilute all essential oils for babies. When in doubt mix a 1:30 blend. This is one part or drop of the essential oil and 30 parts or drops carrier oil, such as YL's V-6™ enhanced vegetable oil complex.

Using oils 'neat' or undiluted will create a tendency for the oil to evaporate more quickly. Using a carrier oil such as V-6 also will create a more sustained effect and reduce possible over-sensitivities especially in newborns.

Sensitivities to YL's essential oils are seen very rarely. Typically, if sensitivities occur, the cause is either that a different brand of chemically adulterated oils were used or because they were used in excess which simply overloaded the system.

Avoid using skin care products, such as shampoos and lotions, which contain petrochemicals that are counteractive to pure, therapeutic-grade essential oils.

Often the following are mentioned in aromatherapy guides as oils to avoid during pregnancy: Basil, Birch, Calamus, Cassia, Cinnamon bark, Hyssop, Idaho Tansy, Lavandin (a form of lavender often sold in stores), Rosemary, Sage and Tarragon. There are a few times throughout this book where a single oil or blend of one of these oils is used. Historically, there have been instances where non-therapeutic-grade essential oils (adulterated, synthetic and of poor quality) have possibly caused a problem during pregnancy. The many moms who have contributed to this book have used all the oils mentioned in the manner suggested without problems because they used the YL brand. The difference is quality.

In her book "Clinical Aromatherapy: Essential Oils in Practice," Jane Buckle, Ph.D., R.N., states "There are no records of abnormal fetuses or aborted fetuses due to the normal use of essential oils, either by inhalation or topical application. There are no records of a few drops of essential oils taken by mouth causing any problem either."

When to seek medical attention

While most of the symptoms in this book are everyday ailments mom can confidently handle at home, it is important to know when to seek medical attention.

The following conditions require immediate attention from a midwife or doctor:

• Vaginal bleeding.

• Arterial bleeding, characterized by spurts with each beat of the heart, bright red in color and usually severe and hard to control.

• Lethargy, weakness and difficulty awakening.

• Stiff neck with headache and inability to touch chin to chest.

• Bulging of the baby's fontanel (soft spot on baby's head).

• Broken bones.

• Dehydration, which includes dry lips with dry mouth and no urination for six hours.

• Severe allergic reactions to bee, wasp or other insect stings, producing swelling of the throat and tongue and difficulty breathing.

• Red streaks on the skin emanating from an infection point, possibly indicating blood poisoning.

• Burns that cover more area than the size of the hand, or second or third degree burns that become infected.

What are essential oils?

*"Every good gift and every perfect gift is from above, and
cometh down from the Father of lights, with whom there is no
variableness, neither shadow of turning." James 1:17*

Essential oils are the aromatic, volatile liquids distilled from plants.
The oil can be obtained from the seeds, roots, an entire shrub,
flowers, leaves and trees. Each plant may contain hundreds of
molecular chemical compounds with names such as terpenes,
sesquiterpenes, phenols and aldehyes, to name a few. The Bible
contains 188 references to the use of essential oils or the plants
from which they are derived.

Essential oils are very complex and currently under much study for
their remarkable benefits to our health. For example, Clary Sage
has 900 different molecules and lavender over 400.

Like all living things essential oils have a frequency or energy level.
Frequency is a measure of the electrical energy that is constant
between two points. Bruce Tainio, founder and president of Infinity
Resources, Inc., in Cheney, Wash., first developed the technology
to measure the frequency of a substance. Plants and their frequencies
will vary from plant to plant.

The majority of plant essential oils are obtained by steam distillation to release the plants' precious oil. Only one company – Young
Living Essential Oils (YL) – has earned my trust and endorsement.
YL's sophisticated and proprietary steam distillation process uses
low heat, proper pressure, precise timing and of course fresh,
properly grown and harvested plants to deliver essential oils with
quality and purity unmatched in today's market.

Here is an example of the importance of precise timing during
distillation. Cypress has 280 known chemical constituents, and all
280 constituents must be present for cypress to have medicinal
and healing potency. If it is distilled for 20 hours, only 20 of the

280 properties are released. If distilled for 26 hours none of the properties are released. Most cypress available on the U.S. market is distilled for about three and a half hours. The correct length of time for distilling cypress is 24 hours, releasing all 280 properties.

Also, think about this: it takes 5000 pounds of rose PETALS to make just one pound of therapeutic-grade rose essential oil. This equates to a truckload of petals. Any rose oil that is inexpensive is basically useless due to synthetic adulteration and will likely pose a health hazard.

YL essential oils go through numerous in-house and independent lab tests and are graded to meet or exceed Association Francaise de Normalisation (AFNOR) standards and International Organization for Standardization (ISO) standards. They are never adulterated, synthetic or chemically enhanced. If they do not make the grade, they are not given the YL label.

Cheap, synthetic, diluted oils are potentially toxic. Therefore, it is very important to use only high-quality essential oils from a trusted source – like right from the farms. YL, the largest producer of therapeutic-grade essential oils in the world, has over 4,500 acres of aromatic farmland where properly grown, harvested, distilled, bottled and blended oils are produced.

The old adage — you get what you pay for — is especially true in the essential oil industry.

How to use essential oils

"All thy garments smell of myrrh, and aloes (sandalwood), and cassia, out of the ivory palaces, whereby they have made thee glad." Psalm 45:8

There are many ways to enjoy essential oils while pregnant, for newborn care and with young children. The symptoms section of this book recommends specific oils to use and the application method.

A general guideline when using essential oils is responses should occur relatively quickly. If nothing happens for a while after applying an oil, try another recommended oil that works in a similar fashion. While humans are the same species, we still are biologically different and therefore will respond differently to natural products, such as essential oils.

Furthermore, some people are more sensitive than others. Because essential oils are highly concentrated natural plant substances, often it is not the amount of essential oil used at any given application, but the natural frequency of the oil that creates powerful results. This is one reason natural remedies differ vastly from Western medicine because the strength of an essential oils comes through their ability to change the body and the emotions getting to the root of the issue, rather than just an isolated single function or symptom.

Regarding dilution, use a carrier oil such as Young Living (YL) Essential Oils' V-6™ enhanced vegetable oil complex, olive oil, almond oil, jojoba oil or other organic plant-based fatty oil. Please note that fatty oils, unlike aromatic oils, can become rancid. Pure aromatic oils stored in a cool, dry place in dark amber or colored glass bottles will not become rancid.

A treadmill will not help someone lose weight if it's not used daily; neither may a person experience the full benefit of essential oils without regular use. The information contained in this book provides detailed instructions for each application.

INHALING

Place two to three drops of the oil in the palm of the hand, rub together gently in a clockwise motion, cup hands over the nose and mouth and inhale slowly for six to eight minutes. Up to three oils may be used at a time. Oils travel through the nasal passages into the lungs and then to every cell in the body and also pass into the brain via the limbic system. Some people experience physical changes, mental alertness, clarity, relaxation, emotional release and much more just by inhaling the oils. Diluting an essential oil for inhaling is not generally necessary. They also can be smelled straight out of the bottle. Inhale slowly and steadily. Do not snort the oil, as the vapors can irritate the nasal passages and, while no harm is done, this can cause temporary discomfort.

Inhaling is reportedly good for headaches, nervous conditions, anxiety, restlessness, energy, stamina, concentration, cardiovascular challenges and respiratory conditions. In fact, aromatherapy is the science of smell and how it affects the body, mind and spirit.

Please note that smelling through inhaling, diffusing and topical application may bring up old memories — some good, some not so good. This is a great time to deal with those negative emotions that may prevent an individual from achieving his or her highest potential by forgetting the past and moving forward.

A Noble Prize for Physiology or Medicine was awarded to Richard Axel, M.D., and Linda Buck, Ph.D., in 2004 for their perceptive discovery of the human genome, specifically the odorants receptors for the sense of smell and the organization of the olfactory system (Nobelprize.org, 2004). The amount of human genome dedicated to smell is many folds larger than any other human genome.

DIFFUSING

YL's cold-air diffuser is highly recommended to most effectively disperse the oil's thousands of molecules into the air. A cold air diffuser does not to harm the molecules; heat changes the chemical structure of the molecules, rendering the medicinal and healing properties ineffective. Place eight to ten drops of oil into the diffuser's well and let it run for about 15 minutes twice per day. The diffuser can be moved from room to room to truly clean the air and make a room smell great. Diffusing may cut the duration of a cold and, in some homes, can actually prevent illness. For example, YL's Thieves blend was tested at Weber State University (1997) for its potent antimicrobial properties. Thieves was found to have a 99.96 percent kill rate against airborne bacteria, viruses, mold and fungi.

When using a humidifier, fill the humidifier with water and then place a tissue or cloth sprinkled with a few drops of oil in front of the escaping vapor. Since essential oils can dissolve petrochemicals (plastics), placing the drops of oil directly into the humidifier may cause it to degrade over time.

TOPICAL

The word neat means to apply the oils without diluting. For instance with a bug bite, simply apply one or two drops of Purification™ oil onto the skin and rub it around. It is recommended to dilute oils for application to small children and babies until skin sensitivity is known. More is not always better with essential oils; they are very powerful by the drop. Only use essential oils in diluted form in the genital area and on mucus linings as some might sting if not diluted with a carrier oil such as YL's V-6 enhanced vegetable oil complex or any vegetable oil.

If an essential oil is applied topically and the skin begins to turn red, itchy or hot, add olive oil or V-6 oil until there is relief. Nothing is wrong; the oil just brought blood to the skin's surface quickly. This also may occur to those in the habit of using chemical cleansers and soaps, cosmetics, lotions and such with synthetic ingredients, which penetrate the dermal layers of the skin. Applying essential oils to these areas may cause skin irritations and can take these toxins deep into the skin. YL offers a variety of all-natural personal care products for people and pets.

Essential oils can be used for all sorts of ear and eye complaints. For the ears: Apply the suggested oil to the outer back area, under the ear lobe and down the throat to relieve an earache. A cotton ball with a few drops of oil tucked in the ear can also relieve earaches. Oils should not be dropped directly into the ear canal.

For the eyes: While oils should never be used directly in the eye, to support optical wellness use oils on the boney area around the eye and across the bridge of the nose. Many people have reported improved eyesight and sty and pinkeye relief, by using essential oils at both full strength or diluted. Though it will not cause damage, if oil is accidentally put in the eye, it will sting for a bit and most likely cause the eye to water. For immediate relief, place a drop of V-6 into the eye to absorb the essential oil. Never rinse with water as oil and water do not mix, and the oil will spread further.

Vita Flex is a special technique similar to reflexology, using essential oils on various pressure points on the bottom of the feet. Some people are surprised at the results achieved by adding oils to the feet. Dilution, even on children, is generally not necessary on the feet. Consult a reference book for complete instructions and to find the various points.

Bath time can be very relaxing with essential oils. Combine one cup Epsom salts with one cup non-refined salt and then add five drops of the oil of choice. Stir to fully spread the oil throughout. Add ½ cup of this mixture to very warm or hot running bath water. Relax and let the cares of the world melt away. Replace the salt with two tablespoons of carrier oil to evenly disperse the oils.

Sitz baths are great for hemorrhoids or stitches after childbirth. Combine three to four drops of essential oils with one tablespoon olive oil and add to warm bath water. Continue to add hot water to keep the bath water warm.

Hand and foot applications also are beneficial. For nails, combine one ounce V-6 oil, with five drops of essential oil, such as myrrh, lemon oil and frankincense. Add this to two cups warm water and let hands or finger tips soak until the water cools. Another application is to bottle the nail oil blend and apply to the nails nightly. For feet, add regular lavender or the awesome St. Maries Lavender™ to ¼ cup Epsom salts to a basin of hot water and soak. For any type of foot or nail fungus, add Melrose™ or Purification.

Compresses often are used to drive oils deep. Select oils, drop into the hand, mix in a clockwise motion and apply to the area. Then cover the area with a warm wet cloth and top that with a warm dry cloth. Leave it on until it is cool.

INFANT MASSAGE
One of the many benefits to infant massage includes promoting bonding. Over the years, baby massage also has shown beneficial in assisting overall growth and development, sound sleep, relaxation and reduced fussiness. Additional benefits include relief from the discomforts of gas, colic and digestive complaints. Improvements in respiratory, circulatory and immune system function also have been reported. Gentle massage, using therapeutic-grade essential oils diluted in high-quality carrier oils, is enjoyable for both baby and mom or dad. Parents find the special quality time with baby develops a special bond and using essential oils to support the baby's health give parents confidence in their ability to respond to the child's needs.

Cross-cultural studies show that babies who are held, massaged, carried, rocked and breastfed, grow into adults that are less aggressive and violent, and more compassionate and cooperative. Recent research shows benefits for premature infants and children with asthma and diabetes. Mothers with postpartum depression have shown improvement after starting infant massage.

Think of the baby massage as a gentle stroking of the body, not the vigorous, deep tissue, Swedish variety. Ideally, both the parent and baby should be in a calm relaxed state. However, massage also can help calm a baby; a fussy child may respond well to a massage with Lavender or Peace & Calming™ oil. This may be before bath or bedtime. It is best to wait at least one hour after the baby's feeding.

For specific instructions on massage oils and blends, see the Massage section of the Symptoms Guide on page 62.

The room should be warm, rather than cool. A temperature of about 78 degrees is good. The baby should lay on his or her back on a padded blanket or towel. The parent can either stand over the baby if using a bed or massage table or sit on the floor with the parent's legs form a diamond shape where the baby can lie with his head cradled in the adult's feet. Leave the diaper on, but uncover the baby's arms, legs and torso. Be sure to remove all jewelry so as not to scratch the baby.

The parent should place four to five drops of the massage oil or blend in his or her hands and rub together to warm both the hands and the oil. Apply the oil with long gentle strokes on the arms, legs and then torso. Make the strokes gentle, but not ticklish. The direction of the massage can be in both directions, but end with stokes toward the heart. In the case of digestive concerns (colic, gas, etc), massage in small circles from the right to the left side of the body – the same direction the colon flows. If massaging the scalp, use small circular motion as if shampooing the baby's hair.

During the massage it is fine to softly talk or pray, hum, sing and/ or play soft music. To further bond with the baby, maintain eye contact during the baby massage.

The massage may last 10 to 30 minutes, depending on the mood of the child and the desired results of the massage. Keep a warm towel or blanket nearby to cover the massaged area and keep baby from becoming chilled.

Massage may be done near or around the naval area and spine, but do not focus on these areas. Every parent is capable of giving his or her baby a wonderful massage. A great way to learn more about baby massage is to find a massage therapist skilled in baby or infant massage to teach specific techniques depending on a child's health challenge.

If gas is an issue, hold the legs under the knees, then gently press the knees up toward his or her tummy. This position can help the baby to expel gas.

Hair and scalp massage can be very helpful for many hair conditions. Select the oils from those mentioned in a reference book and combine ½ tablespoon V-6 oil or wheat germ oil and five to 10 drops of essential oil. Dip finger tips in the oil and massage into scalp. Cover with warm towel for 20 to 30 minutes, then shampoo as normal. The YL shampoo and rinse products are loaded with essential oils for specific hair types. These are very concentrated and will not require as much as previously used products, making them very cost effective. Also, adults and children over 12 may use the essential oils neat to clean scalp and hair.

Another massage technique, exclusive to YL, is the Raindrop Technique (RT). A full explanation can be found in the "Essential Oils Desk Reference" (EODR), ylwisdom.com, or "Reference Guide for using Essential Oils," abundanthealth4u.com. Both are excellent reference books on the use of therapeutic-grade essential oils, with emphasis on the Young Living product line. In a nutshell, RT is a set of specific oils gently applied to the spine and feet. Learn the technique by buying YL's RT kit, which comes with a training DVD and give the whole family the Raindrop experience. Heavily diluted oils can be used for serious health issues in young children. Contact a massage therapist qualified to perform RT on children. The Center for Aromatherapy Research and Education, raindroptraining.com, has a listing of certified instructors who may be able to refer clients to certified RT therapists.

A modified RT can be useful for infants, but the giver should be proficient with general baby massage with the oils before attempting a RT. Parents should meet with a therapist for individualized instruction. The most important aspect is extreme dilution, avoiding the warm compress and no neck involvement. Most moms find that giving a baby a regular massage and then applying the diluted RT oils to the baby's feet provides the desired results.

HOMEMADE OINTMENTS*

Those who do not make their own herbal base should use the Young Living Rose Ointment, a mildly scented essential oil ointment for topical use that is ideally suited for enhancing with more essential oils to create personal blend.

Collect the following:
- Two ounce container of Rose Ointment
- Essential oils based on recipe from Symptom Guide – about 10 drops for two ounces of Rose Ointment. (Do not use more than eight single oils or three blends in these creations unless listed in the recipe.)
- Small stainless steel sauce pan (one cup is ideal)
Label for container
- Optional – smaller jars (such as sanitized baby food jars) for lip balms or for sharing. If using smaller jars (one ounce or 1/4 ounce), mix the melted Rose Ointment and the essential oils in a glass measuring cup to pour into the smaller containers.

1. Scoop two ounces of Rose Ointment into the saucepan.
2. Drop the essential oils from the recipe into the empty Rose Ointment container. (Do not wipe the container clean, just use a blunt knife or spatula to empty most of the contents)
3. Warm the Rose Ointment on medium to high heat until melted, remove from heat and let cool two to five minutes. Move the pan around so to get everything melted on the lowest heat possible.
4. Pour melted Rose Ointment back into its container with the added essential oils. The melted Rose Ointment automatically will mix with the added essential oils.
5. Let sit uncovered until solid; this should take approximately one hour depending on room temperature. Do not place mixture in the

refrigerator or freezer to hasten this process. This will result in a hole in the middle of the jar.

6. Label and use.

Those using Young Living's proprietary Ointment as the base may freely use, share and give away but may not make any for resale.

INTERNAL USAGE

Oral ingestion is safe with nearly every YL essential oil; DO NOT ATTEMPT TO TAKE OTHER BRANDS ORALLY. Put a few drops into an empty capsule, cap and swallow with water. Capsules come in many sizes, with the two most common "0" and "00." These may be purchased at most health food stores or through Young Living. This may be diluted 1:1 with olive oil. It is acceptable to place the oils in a small spoonful of maple syrup, honey or Young Living's Blue Agave or add to almond or rice milk or on a cracker or piece of bread and ingest.

Ingestion is beneficial for intestinal issues, supportive of the immune system, digestion, hormone balancing and a host of other body functions. Keep ingestion to the recommendation or to only three or four drops per day while pregnant or nursing.

Oral care should not be neglected. Noel Claffey, M.Dent.Sc., Dean of the Dublin Dental School and Hospital in Ireland, authored a study titled "Essential oil mouthwashes: a key component in oral health management," which was featured in the Journal of Clinical Periodontology in June 2003. This showed that rinsing with essential oils was better protection against gum disease than flossing. YL carries toothpaste and mouthwash containing the Thieves™ blend. To make mouthwash with different essential oils, combine two to three drops of essential oil in one ounce of purified water; then mix, gargle and either spit or swallow. Also, add a drop of Thieves to the toothbrush for an exhilarating brushing experience, freshening breath for hours.

Retention implants or boluses for vaginal or rectal implanting is largely reserved for more serious health concerns and not recommended while pregnant.

FOOD PREPARATION

Families can have loads of fun preparing food, cooking and making drinks with essential oils. YL's quarterly Lifestyle Magazine features several recipes using the YL oils, plus the company YL offers two cookbooks for healthier essential oil food preparation ideas. Add a drop of cinnamon oil to a batch of oat bran muffins. Put basil and dill in salad dressings and sauces. Blend YL's Blue Agave and lemon oil into iced water and stir for delicious lemonade.

With strong oils, such as oregano, even one drop may be too strong. Take a toothpick, insert in the bottle and then stir into the finished sauce, adding more to taste. It is best if the food is not heated in the oven to retain more than just flavor.

HOUSE CLEANING

Cleaning the non-toxic way with essential oils provides much more than a great smell. Most commercial products contain ingredients that can be harmful to people and pets. For a guide to household toxins, go to sharinggreathealth.com and scroll down to the lower left and click on the Article Library. The "Labels and Household Toxins" handout is one of many useful charts and articles. The very concentrated Thieves Household Cleaner is great for walls, floors, kitchens and baths, baby's room and more. Concentrated for cost effectiveness, when tested at Weber State University this cleaner had a kill rate of 99.96 percent versus bacteria, fungus, mold and viruses. Lemon oil is another great choice; mix it with a little baking soda for a scouring cleaner.

The Material Safety Data Sheet states – "Thieves Household Cleaner. Section V, HEATH AND HAZARD DATA, INGESTION: Ingestion of concentrate is not recommended, but no special precautions are needed. If small amounts are consumed, drink water to get rid of the taste."

• • • • •

Some oils may be photosensitizing, meaning they can cause a sunburn if applied in excess and then exposed to the sun.

Potentially photosensitizing oils include ginger and citrus oils such as lemon, tangerine and orange.

Before using an oil always skin test the oil on a small area of the skin first. For babies and children, the feet are a great place to start, usually undiluted. Start slowly with diluted oils on other areas, using no more than two or three oils at once.

Research into the effectiveness of essential oils is ever increasing. A simple search on the Internet reveals thousands of scientific, peer reviewed articles validating the effectiveness and safety of using essential oils.

Loss of Pregnancy

If you suspect you are having a miscarriage, please consult your health care provider immediately.

A miscarriage is the loss of a pregnancy during the first 20 weeks. It is usually the body's way of ending a pregnancy that has had a difficult start. The loss of a pregnancy can be very hard to accept. A woman may wonder why it happened or blame herself, but a miscarriage is no one's fault. Essential oils such as Trauma Life may be useful for the emotional aspect of losing a child. See the Emotional Support section on page 50 of the Symptoms Guide.

Preventing some miscarriages may be as simple as additional progesterone. Early in pregnancy progesterone is made by the small cyst in the ovary called the corpus luteum. After nine to 10 weeks the placenta should be producing enough progesterone to support the pregnancy. Low levels of progesterone that cause miscarriage usually is thought to be from inadequate production from the corpus luteum. Progesterone medication is safe and relatively inexpensive, but studies proving its effectiveness have not been conclusive. If a woman has experienced a previous miscarriage, she should discuss with her health care provider whether progesterone is likely to help with the next pregnancy.

Many bacterial and viral infections can contribute to a miscarriage, including viral infections, such as the cytomegalovirus, bacterial infections such as chlamydia, mycoplasma and streptococcus, or in rare cases parasitic infection such as toxoplasmosis. Disease, such as undiagnosed diabetes, also may cause a miscarriage. Chronic illnesses, exposure to environmental toxins (such as certain metals), and stress have also been suspect in some miscarriages. Industry employees working with chemicals such as dyes, metals or solvents are at greater risk. Maternal stresses and heavy use of tobacco, caffeine, alcohol and drugs also are potential factors.

Mothers should eat a nutritious diet well before conception and throughout pregnancy. See the Nutrition Guide on page 77. Prior to conception rid the home of harmful chemical toxins (household cleaners, air fresheners, detergents, bath and body care products, etc.). Using essential oil and essential-oil-based products from Young Living Essential Oils, is one way to be confident.

Placenta previa is a pregnancy complication in which the placenta has attached to the uterine wall close to or covering the cervix. If you experience painless bright red bleeding be sure to contact your health care provider immediately.

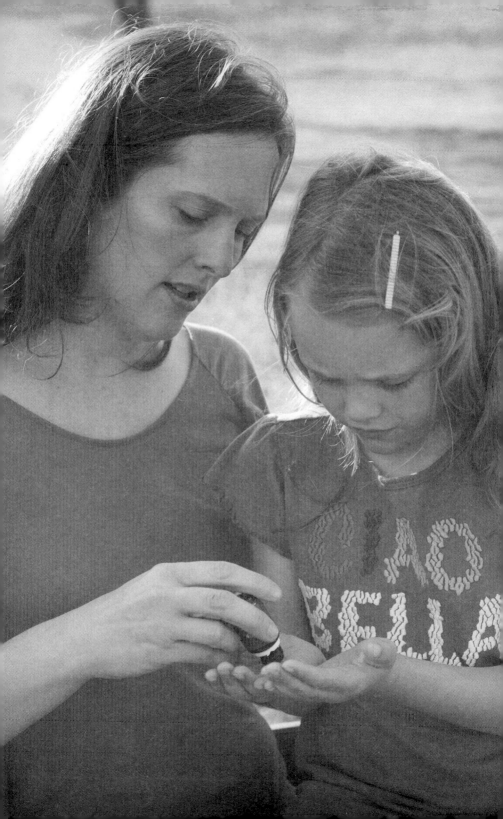

"Thus saith the Lord, thy redeemer, and he who formed thee in the womb: I am the Lord, who has maketh all things; who stretcheth forth the heavens alone; who spreadeth abroad the earth by myself." Isaiah 44:24

The following symptom entries list several possible solutions for pregnant or nursing women and babies or children. Nearly all the suggestions below are an essential oil or a product enhanced with essential oils. From time to time, though, there will be a suggestion concerning a food or herb. Please be selective with products and demand only the very best quality. (See page 14.) The topics included in this guide may be common during a normal pregnancy and childbirth. Certain more serious concerns are not included, as they always require professional medical care and intervention.

Before you begin, remember that you are responsible for your family's health. This guide book suggests holistic remedies, not medical treatment. Most of the symptoms are specific for the baby or child and the mom. In the case when the mother or her little one could have the same condition, such as coughs, and congestion, there may be a "For baby," "For child" and "For mother" suggestion. Typically children up to age five will respond very well with the protocol for babies, but a separate listing "For child" includes applications that children over one year old may respond to quicker. As children grow it is more effective to dilute oils less and apply them more often.

Mothers are free to choose one or use multiple suggestions, as success has been reported with each. If a mother selects more than one essential oil, she should apply the first as directed, then wait 10 minutes. If the desired results are not achieved, then apply the second suggestion. Mothers will no doubt have favorites and should highlight them for future reference.

ACID REFLUX (also see INDIGESTION AND COLIC)

Alkalime™ – Mix one tsp in water in the morning and evening on an empty stomach. Also may be taken after a meal if indigestion causes discomfort.

AFTER BIRTH, CARE FOR AND ANOINTING THE BABY (also see LABOR AND DELIVERY and TRAUMA)

Frankincense – Dilute 1:1 and apply to the whole body as an anointing oil.

Trauma Life™ – Apply wherever the trauma happened or simply on the crown of the head and the feet right after birth.

Valor™ – Dilute in equal parts and apply to feet. Wait five or 10 minutes before using another oil.

Brain Power™, Joy™ and **Peace & Calming™** – Dilute in equal parts and use as a massage oil. Apply to feet and all over the body, including the head.

Lavender – Dilute in equal parts and apply to feet for relaxation when needed.

Myrrh – Dilute 1:1 and apply to the whole body as an anointing oil.

Mix any oil of choice with 30 drops to one ounce carrier oil and apply on abdomen.

AFTER BIRTH CARE FOR MOM

Clara Derm™ Spray – Apply as needed on vaginal area.

Gentle Baby™ – Place two to four drops on abdominal area.

ALLERGIES

For everyone:

Lavender, R.C.™ and **eucalyptus radiata** – Diffuse 20 to 30 minutes twice per day or as needed.

For child over two-years-old:

Eucalyptus radiata – Same as above for mom.

Lavender – Ingest one drop in a teaspoon of honey or YL's Blue Agave once or twice per day.

For mother:

Eucalyptus radiata – Put one drop or less drop on the pinky finger and swab the inside of the nose, but not deeply.

Lavender – Put five drops in a capsule and ingest between meals.

Lavender has been working wonderfully for my allergies. I almost can't believe the difference! ~ April

AUTISM

Many children diagnosed with autism and related disorder symptoms improve with diet change and the use of certain essential oils. Reducing high glycemic, non-nutritive foods with wholesome choices also is quite beneficial. The book *Nutrition 101: Choose Life!* guides families to better, more wholesome eating habits that will benefit all family members. See page 101 for ordering information.

KidScents MightyZymes – Use as directed on bottle.

KidScents MightyVites – Use as directed on bottle.

NingXia Red – Drink one to two ounces per day. Dilute in glass of water, if preferred. This is an excellent source of vitamins and minerals, anti-oxidants and glutathione, which many autistic children are deficient in.

Brain Power, Frankincense, Clarity, Peace & Calming, Idaho Balsam Fir, Valor, Cedarwood and **Sandalwood** – Diffuse any and all. May also have the child apply the oil to the scalp and wear as perfume.

In cases where heavy metals (mercury) is suspect:

Juva Cleanse® – Apply to the bottom of feet at bedtime. Take one or two drops in a capsule or in rice milk twice daily for three months. Immediately remove all chemically laden body care and household cleaning products from the home.

"My son Noah, a five-year-old diagnosed with autisim, could not converse with us; he just repeated phrases he'd heard. In May, we made the commitment to give him three MightyZymes each day, every day. By the end of June, he burst out of his shell. He began talking in a conversational method and asking and answering questions. He wanted us with him, to play with him, to watch movies with him and read to him. I believe that through YL's MightyZymes and essential oils, our Heavenly Father has released our child from many of the daiyl struggles of autism." ~ Evon (Read the complete testimony on page 97.)

35

BABY ACNE

This usually occurs on the cheeks and sometimes on the forehead, chin and back. Milia are tiny bumps that appear on the face at birth and disappear within a few weeks, and they're unrelated to acne. If the irritation is more rashy or scaly than pimply or it appears elsewhere on the body, the baby may have another condition, such as cradle cap or eczema.

Lavender and **Melrose™** – One drop of each dilute 1:1 and apply to affected areas of skin, and be careful to avoid eyes and mouth.

BACK PAIN (also see MUSCULAR PAIN)

PanAway™ – Apply directly or diluted 1:1 on the area of pain.
Valor – Apply directly on the area.
Aroma Siez™ – Apply directly on the area.
Deep Relief™ roll-on – Apply directly on area of discomfort.

BATHING BABY

Use only a mild bath gel or soap on a new baby.
KidScents Bath Gel™ – Follow instructions on the bottle.

BED WETTING

Melrose – Apply neat over the bladder
Omega Blue™ – Pierce a capsule and squeeze the contents into a spoon of YL's Blue Agave, apple sauce or rice milk and consume with evening meal. Omega Blue is available only in the core supplements pack. OmegaGize is a formula for adults.
Peace & Calming and **Valor** – Apply to bottom of feet at bedtime.

Remove all carbonated beverages completely as these are acid forming and may irritate the kidneys and bladder, exacerbating this condition. Stop all fluids two hours before bedtime.

> "My daughter started taking one Omega Blue capsule each day to help her unexplained bed wetting, a problem she'd dealt with since she was a toddler. Beginning the day she started taking Omega Blue, she has never wet the bed again; it was that effective" ~ Sera

BLEEDING, internal for mother:

If bleeding vaginally, consult with a midwife or doctor immediately

Shock Tea – For this home remedy, use one cup warm water, three tablespoons apple cider vinegar and one teaspoon cayenne pepper and three tablespoons honey (optional). Stir all together and drink with a straw.

Helichrysum - Put 10 drops in a "00" capsule and seek medical attention.

Trauma Life – Apply externally to the wrists and inhale to reduce the stress of the issue.

BLEEDING, external

Tsuga – Apply externally on location.

Geranium – Apply one to two drops directly for any bleeding around umbilical cord/belly button. This may be diluted.

Rose Ointment – Apply topically to the area.

Helichrysum - Apply one to two drops helichrysum to the skin where the bleeding is happening. Apply slight pressure and repeat if needed.

NOTE: With bleeding on the skin wash with clean cool water and then cover with a damp gauze or cloth and apply pressure. Apply Tsuga or Helichrysum oil to the area and recover. Check in five to 10 minutes. If stitches are required, go to the nearest medical facility. In almost all cases of minor bleeding, the Tsuga oil and then a small amount of Rose Ointment is all that is required.

BLOOD PRESSURE/HYPERTENSION

Preeclampsia, also known as pregnancy-induced hypertension (PIH), is a form of high blood pressure occurring only during pregnancy.

Aroma Life™ – Apply one or two drops on the heart area and inner wrist to normalize low blood pressure. Also inhale.

Clary Sage – Apply one or two drops on the heart area and inner wrist to lower and normalize blood pressure.

NingXia Red™ – Drink one to two ounces a day to normalize.

Lavender – Inhale every five minutes until desired results. Ingesting one drop on tongue may lower blood pressure.

BLOOD SUGAR (see GESTATIONAL DIABETES)

BONDING WITH BABY
Gentle Baby – Apply one or two drops on the pregnant belly.
Joy – Inhale or apply one or two drops to breasts, but not on nipples, prior to nursing.

"I used Joy to help relieve stress and promote additional bonding because my daughter was premature and spent a week in the neonatal intensive care unit. As a toddler, anytime she is fussy or agitated, I have her inhale Joy, apply it to her like perfume and say 'the joy of the Lord is our strength.'" ~ Laura

BREAST INFECTION/ MASTITIS/MILK FEVER
This can occur if breast are not emptied completely or when milk ducts get clogged or if breast feeding is abruptly stopped.
Geranium (one drop), **Lavender** (one drop) and (two drops) – Combine oils in 1.5 pints cold water, dip washcloth into it, squeeze excess water out and apply on breast as a cold compress. Repeat as frequently as each hour during the day.
If fever is associated:
Eucalyptus globulus – Add five drops to ½ teaspoon sea salt to a basin of warm water and soak feet. Repeat as frequently as each hour during the day.
Melrose – Apply a warm compress to a clogged milk duct.

BREECH BABIES
When the baby has not turned to be vertex (head down) for labor and delivery, but is presenting bottom first, the position is termed breech.
Peppermint – Apply to the abdomen. (See midwife testimony on page 84.)
Myrrh – Apply several drops to the belly and rub them into the skin. Repeating the application may be needed.

CESAREAN/C-SECTION

This is a surgical procedure where an incision through the abdomen and uterus is used to extract the baby.

Rose – One drop on location may assist in releasing emotional trauma and is rejuvenating to the skin/tissue.

Helichrysum – One drop on location heals tissue trauma and stops bleeding.

Lavender – Liberally apply on location to prevent scaring and promote skin healing.

Believe™ – One drop diluted on the area for wound healing.

Trauma Life – One drop on location covers a large terrain of application.

CHICKEN POX

Chicken pox, or Herpes zoster, is related to the Herpes simplex virus. Unlike shingles - what herpes zoster is called when it manifests in adults - chicken pox is highly contagious.

ClaraDerm Spray – Spray on rash to relieve itching.

Australlan Blue, Roman Chamomlle, Lavender, Melrose and **Ravensara** – Apply one drop of each to the bottom of the feet three times daily at onset.

NingXia Red – Drink one ounce daily

Ravensara– Dilute 1:1 with V-6 and dab on spots.

Raindrop Technique – Refer to the Essential Oils Desk Reference for instructions on this technique, which is very useful for all types of viral conditions including chicken pox, shingles and measles.

CIRCULATION

Cypress, Helichrysum and **Tangerine oil** – Combine a couple of drops of each with several drops of a carrier oil and massage legs every day.

NingXia Red – Drink one ounce twice a day.

Ortho Ease® massage oil – Apply to restless legs.

Omega Blue or **OmegaGize** – Take one to four capsules daily as directed on bottle.

CIRCUMCISION
Rose Ointment– Apply topically with each diaper change to prevent healing area from sticking to diaper.
Animal Scents Ointment– Apply topically, as directed above. Despite the name, Animal Scents Ointment works well for humans too.

COLD SORE
Cold Sore Ointment – Use the ingredients below and follow the instructions on page 26 to create this ointment. Apply to the cold sore multiple times a day.
Lavender (two drops)
Melissa (two drops)
Melrose (two drops)
Sandalwood (two drops)
Ravensara (one drop)
Thyme (one drop)

COLIC
This is when an infant has episodes of crying and irritability with what appears to be abdominal pain. Nursing mothers should examine their diet for offending foods and avoid caffeine, foods with high fat content and spicy foods that may be too harsh for the baby.
Roman Chamomile – Place one drop in bowl of warm water and compress on baby's belly.
Dill – Place one drop in one tablespoon of either V-6 oil or sweet almond oil and rub on the middle of the baby's back in circular, clockwise motions.
Di-Gize™ – Dilute one drop in one teaspoon olive oil rubbed on the baby's abdomen.

CONGESTION (also see COUGHING and RESPIRATORY INFECTION)
Eucalyptus globulus, Eucalyptus radiata, R.C. or **Rosemary** – Diffuse all to decongest.

"Not long after my son was born, my family dealt with a nasty upper respiratory visur with major congestion and a croupy coughing. Of course, we all increased our NingXia Red doses up to three to six ounces a day. My daughters, husband and I all took three to five Inner Defense capsules a day, and I diffused and applied lots of R.C. to our chests, necks and feet helping us get rid of it in about half the time it would have normally taken. However, my five-week-old came down with a low fever and had some congestion which I knew was pretty serious for a newborn. I rubbed R.C., diluted 1:1 with V-6 oil, all over his chest and bottoms of his feet every two hours or so and applied lavender to the bridge of his nose for a blocked tear duct. As I was praying over him, I felt led to apply Frankincense all over his body, around the outside of his eyes, and over his sinuses. I also diluted some Thieves 1:1 and rubbed it on the bottom of his feet. The next day, his fever was gone, the congestion was cleared, and even the blocked tear duct was open and the infection in his eye was totally cleared up!" ~ Sera

CONTRACTIONS (see LABOR)

CONSTIPATION
FOR BABY AND CHILD:
KidScents MightyVites™ and **KidScents MightZyme** – For children who are eating solids, use as directed on bottle.
Peppermint – Dilute one or two drops and apply to the abdomen and rub in circular, clockwise motions.
Di-Gize – Apply diluted 1:1 or neat to lower abdomen and bottom of the feet.
Fennel – Apply neat to bottom of the feet in the center and heel area.
FOR MOTHER:
Life 5 Probiotic™ – This probiotic supplement may assist in proper bowel function. Use as directed on bottle.
Comfortone™ – If tendency toward constipation exists, comfortone capsules before breakfast and bedtime may provide relief. Start with one capsule and increase daily as needed.

Follow appropriate nutrition to prevent constipation. (See Nutrition Guide on page 77.) Drink eight or more eight-ounce glasses of distilled water throughout the day for best results. Do not begin taking Comfortone in the last trimester unless instructed by your health care provider.

ICP™ – Mix two teaspoons with at least eight ounces of fresh juice or water and drink daily. This contains advanced fibers that scour the colon; increased fiber leads to better bowel formation and movement. Do not take more than one teaspoon per day after third month.

Essentialzyme™ – One to three capsules before meals to improve digestion, which is challenged in general during pregnancy.

Balance Complete™ – Add two scoops to eight to ten ounces of cold water with breakfast and/or lunch.

NingXia Red – Two to three ounces daily.

COUGHING (also see RESPIRATORY INFECTION and WHOOPING COUGH)

Lemon oil and **Purification™** – Diffuse several drops of either or both about 15 to 20 minutes in the bedroom before bedtime.

Lemon oil – Ingest one or two drops in a teaspoon of Grade B Maple Syrup or YL's Blue Agave.

Thieves – Place one to two drops on the bottom of the feet.

Peace & Calming – Place a few drops on the chest mixed with a few drops of carrier oil.

Homemade onion and garlic poultice:
   One small onion diced into large chunks
   One teaspoon fresh garlic, minced
   Two tablespoons olive oil

Place the diced onion in a glass baking dish and heat in the oven at 350°F for about 20 minutes, or until the onion begins to be clear and slimy. Remove from oven and pour onion into a clean bowl. Add garlic and olive oil. Let cool until warm, but not hot. Strain the oil into a clean bowl to remove the chunks. Place the oil on the baby's chest, cover with a warm wet wash cloth. Now cover with another dry wash cloth or towel. Let poultice remain on chest and allow baby to rest for two hours. Remove the poultice.

> "When Joshua was 10 months old, he got a severe upper respiratory virus. I did not have any Young Living essential oils at the time, so that morning I tried the onion and garlic poultice. After the first application, the congestion started breaking up, and he was having productive coughs. Then, a few hours later, I did it again. By that night, his lungs were totally clear, and he slept great!" ~ Sera

CRADLE CAP

The medical term is seborrheic dermatitis, and it describes the inflammation in the upper layers of the skin, causing scales on the scalp, face and occasionally other areas. This condition may be due to low intake of biotin in the mothers diet. Refer to page 101 the author's book *Nutrition 101: Choose Life!* for information of obtaining biotin from food.

Lavender – Dilute or use neat on affected area.

Melrose – Dilute or use neat on affected area.

Rose ointment - Apply to the scalp. It also may be combined with a drop of either or both of the oils listed above.

CRYING BABY

Peace & Calming – Apply neat to the feet and back of neck. Also have the baby smell the oil from mom or dad's hands.

Lavender and **Joy** – Have the baby smell the oil from an adult's hands.

> "When my newborn is crying and I know he is not hungry, wet, or sleepy, I hold different oils up to his nose for him to smell. Most of the time, he stops crying as he is experiencing this new smell and even settles down as if he forgot why he was crying. By experimenting like this, I have found that one of his favorites is lavender. It really helps to calm him." ~ Sera

DETOXIFYING

It is not the time to embark on an aggressive cleanse during pregnancy and while nursing. Once a baby is weaned or at least only nursing a few times per day is generally the time when a mother can begin more aggressive cleanse. Until then it is best to drink one to two servings of Balance Complete daily (as a snack, not meal replacement); drink Green Smoothies (see page 80 for the recipe); and drink NingXia Red to maintain mild nourishing cleanse. Also refer to the section on Nutrition Guide on page 77.

DIAPER PAILS (see House Cleaning on page 28)

Thieves Household Cleaner™ can help keep the diaper pail sanitized and smelling fresh for moms using cloth diapers. In one pint of cool water add one capful of Thieves Household Cleaner. Pour into the bottom of the clean diaper pail.

DIAPER RASH

Avoid commercial products that contain irritants such as talc and mineral oil.

Gentle Baby – Dilute 1:30 with YL V-6 or almond oil and apply on location.

Tender Tush™ ointment – Apply topically.

Animal Scents™ ointment – Apply topically.

Rose ointment – Apply topically.

Diaper ointment recipe – Use the ingredients below and follow the instructions on page 26 to create this ointment. Apply multiple times a day.

- **Gentle Baby** (four drops)
- **Lavender** (two drops)
- **German Chamomile** (two drops)
- **Cypress** (one drop)
- **Melrose** (one drop)

Baby powder alternative – Mix two tablespoons of cornstarch with five drops of either Lavender, Rose or Gentle Baby essential oil. Sift together several times until well blended. Store in a tightly sealed container.

Baby oil alternative – Mix two tablespoons of hazelnut oil, olive oil or V-6 oil with five drops **Lavender** or **Gentle Baby**. Store in a tightly sealed container.

Homemade baby wipes

Take a roll of natural paper towels, which typically are brown in color and made from recycled paper and contain no chemicals, just 100 percent cotton/natural fibers. Cut the roll in half using a serrated knife. Obtain a clean round container with a tight fitting lid that will hold the half roll. Flatten the roll and then remove the inner cardboard core. Place the half roll in the container. In a separate bowl, add:

  2 cups distilled or boiled bottled water that has cooled to room temperature

  2 Tbls. Young Living Lavender Shampoo or KidScents shampoo

  2 Tbls. V-6 mixing oil blend

  5 drops of any Young Living Essential Oil of choice, such as **Lavender**, **Gentle Baby**, **Sandalwood**, or **Frankincense**.

(Adding essential oils is optional because the Young Living shampoos contain therapeutic-grade essential oils.)

Whisk the mixture together well and pour over the flattened roll in the container. Cover and let sit overnight to absorb all the liquid. When ready to use, open container and pull a wipe from the center, tear off and use. Close lid securely between uses to avoid drying out. If wipes become dry, add a few tablespoons of sterile water to re-hydrate. Only use the Young Living brand of essential oils.

"My three month old had a severe diaper rash. I tried all the normal ointments and was getting no where. One day I put some Bert's Bees on him, and he started screaming. I put him in the bathtub and washed him off and decided to apply some Tender Tush. He started laughing at me as I applied it! The rash was gone the next day!" ~ Beverly

DIARRHEA

These suggestions may be used proactively and reactively for all members of the family. In general for babies and children, apply one to two drops over the abdomen. Oral applications are for adults.

Di-Gize – Apply one to two drops over abdomen. In addition, adults may put two drops in water to sip on.

Lavender and **Basil** – Apply one drop of each over abdomen to calm stress induced by diarrhea (**Lavender**, **Basil**, **Cypress**, **Roman chamomile** and **Eucalyptus** are anti-spasmodic.)

Peppermint – One drop orally.

Ledum – Apply one to two drops over abdomen and take one drop orally.

ICP – Place a few teaspoons in water to absorb excess water in the colon.

Inner Defense – Take one capsule per day if a stomach bug is the possible cause.

Life 5 – Take one or two capsules daily to establish the good gut flora in the system.

Geranium, **Sandalwood** and **Roman Chamomile** – Apply one to two drops applied over abdomen.

DIETARY REGIMEN DURING PREGNANCY (see NUTRITION GUIDE on page 77)

NingXia Red – Two to three ounces daily.

Core Supplements™ – Take daily as directed.

Omega Blue or **OmegaGize** – Take one to four capsules daily as directed on bottle.

Pure water – Ingest half body weight in ounces, plus an additional 20 ounces to avoid swelling in hands, legs and feet. This also helps prevent nausea.

Pure Protein Complete™ – Take as directed for extra protein needs, especially for breakfast. Eat lots of fresh vegetables and fruit.

DILATION, if delayed and the health adviser or midwife recommends encouraging dilation

Clary Sage – Massage around the ankle bone or ingest one drop every 15 minutes until dilation begins. Other moms have taken six drops and then take a wait-and-see attitude and reassess after four or five hours. Monitor over the next couple hours. Then repeat if necessary. Do not try to force the delivery.

EAR INFECTIONS

Ledum or **Melrose** – Dilute 1:10 and apply one or two drops all around on the outer ear, down the neck and on the feet several times daily.

Thieves – Apply one or two drops to the feet.

FOR EXTREME CASES ONLY** – As mentioned previously on page 22, it is not recommended to place essential oils directly into the ear canal. There is an exception, but only under the following guidelines: restricintg the use of a pacifier; eliminating all milk consumption, including raw cow or goat; making sure the bowels are working properly, meaning two to three times daily; and the above mentioned oils on the outer ear fail to relieve the pain and discomfort. Use the following recipes with confidence making no substitutions or exceptions for safety and effectiveness. Mix the following in an ¼ ounce or less dropper bottle:

V-6 or first cold press olive oil (10 drops)

Lavender (one drop)

Melrose (one drop)

Use one drop of this mix in each ear one to three times per day. It is rarely needed beyond one day.

FOR AGES TWO AND UP (the same application can be used with the following increases):

10 drops V-6 oil

St. Marie's Lavender (two drops)

Melrose (two drops)

"My six month old got a really bad ear infection. We took him to the doctor and after he went through three rounds of antibiotics, the pediatrician finally suggested an antibiotic injection. I drew the line there, and she said then we would have to go to an Ear, Nose and Throat specialist and get tubes put in his ears. The ENT could not see us for two weeks, so we called a naturopath we had recently meet and asked her what we could do. By now this infection had been going on for a couple of months and was only getting worse. She told us to remove dairy from his diet, rub ledum below his ear and down his neck, rub Thieves on his feet and apply colloidal silver in his ear. When we went to the ENT two weeks later he looked in his ears and said there was no sign of infection. He asked what we had done and of course, in his mind, none of it made any difference. I knew that the oils were what killed this infection." ~ Beverly

"My six-month-old was cranky and pulling on her ears so I used the Melrose blend in her ear several times a day. I would also applied Ledum in a downward motion from her ear to her chin line. She was having a hard time sleeping and was congested as well so I had her at an incline. After putting the oil in her ears with a teeny bit of cotton ball, she slept for hours and was not cranky. I have now learned if I don't eat much dairy while nursing, we can avoid any congestion and ear problems with her. ~ Jeanette

"Our friends were planning to fly again with their two-year-old daughter and did not want to relive a previous flight when she was very agitated and disruptive. They used Peace & Calming prior to the flight, and the child slept through the night for the first time in weeks. During the flight, the child was calm and the Melrose helped alleviate any pressure she and her mom experienced during takeoff and landing." ~ Laura

ECZEMA/DERMATITIS

This is a general term encompassing various inflamed skin conditions. Although it may look different from person to person, it is most often characterized by dry, red, extremely itchy patches on the skin. In infants, eczema typically occurs on the forehead, cheeks, forearms, legs, scalp and neck. In children and adults, it typically occurs on the face, neck, and the insides of the elbows, knees and ankles.

Lavender and **Melrose** – Place two drops in the palm, stir to mix and apply neat on the affected area.

Tender Tush – Apply like lotion all over the skin.

Detoxzyme®️ or Allerzyme™️ – Empty contents of one capsule in food. These have been used on young children who are eating and not nursing.

Lemon oil – Apply neat on the affected area.

Lavender and **Rose Ointment** – Apply a few drops lavender and then top with Rose Ointment.

Lavender Hand and Body Lotion – Slather on the skin.

Irritated skin ointment – Use the ingredients below and follow the instructions on page 26 to create this ointment. Apply as needed.

> **Lavender** (two drops)
> **German Chamomile** (one drop)
> **Cistus** (one drop)
> **Palmarosa** (three drops)
> **Geranium** (two drops)
> **Helichrysm** (one drop)

EDEMA/WATER RETENTION

This includes swelling usually in the legs, feet and ankles.

Cypress and **Tangerine oil** – Add one drop of each to drinking water. Repeat several times a day.

NingXia Red – Drink one to two additional ounces daily.

Water Retention Massage Oil Blend:

> **Tangerine oil** (two drops)
> **Lemon oil** (one drop)
> **Cypress** (four drops)
> **Lavender** (four drops)
> **Geranium** (three drops)

Mix oils into two and ½ tablespoon almond oil, ½ tablespoon jojoba oil and one **Evening Primrose** carrier oil capsule (approximately 10 drops). This can be used all throughout pregnancy. Relax on the sofa with legs raised on pillows. Apply the oils to feet, ankles and legs, massaging toward the heart to help circulation. Husbands usually need to help apply this blend.

EMOTIONAL SUPPORT (also see FEAR, PANIC, POSTPARTUM DEPRESSION, SELF-LOVE, SELF-ESTEEM and TRAUMA)

Forgiveness™ – Diffuse or apply one to two drops to help release the past.

Present Time™ – Diffuse or apply one to two drops to stay focused on the now.

Surrender™ – Diffuse or apply one to two drops to support in releasing negative emotions.

Peace & Calming or **Stress Away roll on**– Apply on wrist and around ears and neck. Rest, relaxation and the ability to think clearly will return. Smelling good will help a mom feel pretty.

ENERGY INCREASE

En-R-Gee™ – Apply one drop on the back, at the approximate location of each kidney, and one drop over the left and right ribs and/or on bottom of both feet.

Peppermint – Apply one drop in the same locations as above or on the neck area. Ingest a drop of peppermint in drinking water daily.

Lemon and **Grapefruit oils** – A few drops in drinking water. Also inhale.

FOR CHILD AND MOTHER:

NingXia Red – Drink three to six ounces per day, spread throughout the day. Some people are so energized by NingXia Red that they cannot drink it after 4 p.m. because it provides extra energy that prolongs their bed time.

EPISIOTOMY (also see PERINEUM CARE)

This is a small incision to further open the perineum to allow more room for the baby to be delivered. They often require stitches to aid in healing.

Peace & Calming – Diffuse during labor.

Lavender – Add several drops to bath water at birth or diffuse it in the room.

Lavaderm Cooling Mist™ – Spray the area after birth.

Clara Derm Spray™ – Apply as needed for six weeks prior to birth and after.

EYE CONDITIONS (clogged tear ducts, pinkeye and sty)

Mites can adhere to the eyelashes of adults and children and cause vision and eye problems.

Lavender – Apply one drop to bridge of the nose and on the bone surrounding the eye, careful to avoid the eye. This is good for clogged tear ducts, pinkeye and sties.

Melaleuca alternifolia (tea tree) – Mix two drops with one ounce tepid water. Close the eye and wash the eye lids with a cotton ball dipped into the solution. Use a new cotton ball each time. Rinse with cool water, pat dry.

Eye support blend:

  Olive Oil (20 drops)
  Lavender (20 drops)
  Melrose (20 drops)
  Frankincense (10 drops)

Combine in a small dropper bottle. Place one drop on a clean index finger, rub together with the other index finger. Gently apply around the boney part of the eye. May also be placed on the toe reflex point.

FEAR (also see EMOTIONAL SUPPORT)

FOR BABY OR CHILD:

Valor – Apply or roll-on to back of neck, on feet and inhale daily as needed.

FOR MOM:

  Valor, Surrender and **Believe** – Wear as a perfume and inhale as needed to help with courage and focus and to dispel any fears associated with pregnancy and childbirth.

"I used Present Time and Surrender to help me with my fear to push, and it was amazing how fast Jack came!"
~ Beverly

FEVER

FOR BABY:

Peppermint – Dilute 1:1 and apply to the navel.

Lavender – Apply one or two drops to the bottom of the feet.

Thieves – Apply one or two drops to the bottom of the feet.

FOR CHILD:

Peppermint – Apply neat to the navel.

Lavender or **Thieves** – Apply one or two drops to the bottom of the feet hourly.

NingXia Red – one ounce every couple of hours.

FOR MOM, SAME AS CHILD PLUS:

Inner Defense™ – one capsule or more daily.

FORMULA ENHANCERS

Many moms are faced with a dilemma: either their milk supply is not sufficient for the baby (even after using the milk-boosting suggestions in on page 60) or they are not breast feeding and want to supplement traditional formula. The following enhancers are not to be used in lieu of regular formula, but may be used with breastfeeding or with regular formula, especially when milk supply is low or the baby is not gaining weight properly.

Enhancer recipe:

Six ounces of purified water

One half scoop of **Power Meal** (amino acid and nutrient rich powder)

One half scoop of **Pure Protein** (whey-based powder that contains 13 grams of protein per serving)

One teaspoon to one tablespoon **NingXia Red**

Mix well in a blender. This also may be mixed with goats milk or rice milk. Use twice daily.

FUNGAL INFECTIONS

These may appear on the skin, between toes or folds of skin.

Eucalyptus blue – Apply one drop neat on the area. Dilution is acceptable, but this oil typically causes no skin sensitivities.

Athletes Foot ointment – Use the ingredients below and follow the instructions on page 26 to create this ointment. Apply to clean feet and toes twice daily.

Abundance (two drops)

Melrose (two drops)

Thieves (one drop)

FOR MOTHER:

Female Salve – Use the ingredients below and follow the instructions on page 26 to create this ointment. It may be used topically or as an insertion when pregnant or nursing for itching, genital herpes, candida and infections.

Gentle Baby (three drops)
3 Wise Men (three drops)
Patchouli (three drops)

GESTATIONAL DIABETES – (also see NUTRITION GUIDE on page 77)

This refers to pregnant women who have never had diabetes, but whose blood sugar levels rise during pregnancy. As the baby develops hormones from the placenta, this can block the action of the mother's insulin in her body and make it hard for the mother's body to use insulin. This condition requires monitoring by a health professional to avoid serious complications for mother and baby. Avoid highly processed food, especially refined white flour and white sugar foods.

NingXia Red – Drink three ounces over the course of a day.
Pure Protein Complete or **Power Meal** – Take one to two servings per day between meals.
Ocotea – Place two drops in ½ ounce NingXia Red in the morning, mid afternoon and before bedtime.
For a healthy snack, make the green smoothies on page 80.

I tested positive for gestational diabetes with my first child and then again with my fourth. I managed to control it with diet during my first pregnancy. However, with my fourth, I was so frustrated and had to almost starve myself to keep my sugars down. I was absolutely fearful that I would have to go on insulin. Then I got my Ningxia Red. I started taking one ounce three times a day, following each meal. Within three to four days I noticed a dramatic difference. My sugars were less than 120 almost all the time. I was usually high once or twice a week after starting NingXia Red, but when I was high it was only in the 130's not the 180's. After a week I noticed that I was able to eat larger portions and still maintain my sugars within range. That is awesome when you are pregnant and hungry almost all the time! I had a healthy, full-term, eight pound baby girl with zero complications. Praise God! ~ Becky, R.N.

GROUP BETA STREP

The bacteria Group B Streptococcus (GBS) has been identified as the number one cause of life-threatening infections in newborns. Normally found in 40 percent of all healthy women, those who test positive for GBS are said to be colonized. This should not be confused with Group A Streptococcus, which causes strep throat.

Thieves – Apply three drops on soles of feet morning and night.
Valor – Apply five drops distributed along the spine, morning and night.
Inner Defense – Take three to five capsules daily.
Life 5 Probiotic – Take one capsule each evening. This is included in the Core Supplements.

HAND-FOOT-AND-MOUTH DISEASE

This is a common childhood illness which may feature mouth sores, fever and a rash. It may be caused by a variety of viruses in the Enterovirus family, specifically coxsackievirus A16. This condition is not to be confused with foot and mouth disease, which infects cattle and is rare in humans.

Thieves, **Mountain Savory**™ or **Purification** – Dilute or apply two or three drops neat on the feet and spine several times throughout the day. These oils also may be alternated.

A few days before we were going out of town to see family, I noticed red bumps/blisters on my son's feet. Because he had slept terribly the night before, I immediately suspected hand-foot-and-mouth disease. He did not have blisters on his hands or mouth, nor did he have a fever or other symptoms. I chalked it up to teething. By lunchtime, he had developed the blisters on his hands. I still didn't see any in his mouth, but I knew it had to be the virus especially when he wouldn't eat solids for dinner that night. I began to apply Thieves on his feet and spine. I alternated with Mountain Savory and Purification. Just an hour or so after applying the Purification, I tried to show the bumps to my mom, and I could only find two! I kept applying the Purification at every diaper change on Monday and continued as we traveled Tuesday.

By Wednesday, the bumps we gone from his hands and only red spots remained on his feet! He never seemed to have the fever, but the Purification really seemed to have shortened the duration of the virus! ~ Wendy

HEADACHES

Lavender – Place a drop on temples, back of neck, across forehead and on the painful location. Also inhale.

Frankincense – Place a drop on temples, back of neck, across forehead and on the painful location. Also inhale.

Peppermint – Place a drop on temples, back of neck, across forehead and on the painful location. Also inhale.

Roman Chamomile – Place a drop or less on temples, back of neck, across forehead and on the painful location. Also inhale. NOTE: Many ladies like to place one drop peppermint, one drop lavender and one drop Frankincense in the palm of the hands, and mix in a clockwise motion. Rub the hands together, cup over nose and mouth and hale.

HEART BURN (see also ACID REFLUX)

Peppermint – Ingest one drop or apply one to two drops on the chest when needed.

Di-Gize – Apply three to four drops directly on the mother's belly. May also ingest one to drop orally.

A combination of the above works best.

NingXia Red – Sip on as needed.

AlkaLime – Dissolve one teaspoon in four ounces of water and drink early morning and late evening.

HEMORRHOIDS

Rose Ointment – Apply topically.

Balance Complete – Eat plenty of nutritious fiber. Balance Complete is a great high-fiber, high-protein, nutritionally dense drink mix and is delicious in smoothies.

Hemorrhoid Relief Blend – Combine the following oils with two to four drops of V-6 oil and apply to the area.

Peppermint (one drop)

Helichrysum (two drops)
Geranium (two drops)
Cypress (two drops)

Hemorrhoid ointment #1 – Use the ingredients below and follow the instructions on page 26 to create this ointment. Apply until problem solved.

Cypress (three drops)
Cistus (two drops)
Basil (three drops)
Spikenard (one drop)
Wintergreen (one drop)

Hemorrhoid ointment #2 – Use the ingredients below and follow the instructions on page 26 to create this ointment. Apply until problem solved.

Cypress (four drops)
Myrtle (two drops)
Myrrh (two drops)
Roman Chamomile (two drops)

"After Jack's birth I had a hemorrhoid that was very uncomfortable. I tried all the normal stuff – more fiber, water, etc. – and just could not get it to go away. Finally, I put together this blend of one drop peppermint, two drops helichrysum and two drops cypress and a couple drops of V-6 oil. In less than a week it was completely gone!" ~ Beverly

INDIGESTION
FOR BABY AND CHILD:

Di-Gize – Apply a drop on the belly, diluted 1:1.

Peppermint – Apply a drop on the bottom of the feet diluted 1:10. This will aid digestion and help to prevent colic.

FOR MOTHER:

Peppermint – Place one drop on the tongue.

Alkalime – Put one teaspoon in water in the morning and evening on an empty stomach, may take after a meal if indigestion is severe.

Essentialzyme – Take two tablets with a meal to aid in digestion.

INSECT BITES

Purification - Apply one drop on a bite. For prevention, apply one to two drops daily on the bottom of feet.

Insect Repellent Spray – Gentle enough for babies. For every four ounces of distilled water add five drops of **Purification** and five drops of **Peppermint**.

"I have a few kids that swell up immediately with any kind of insect bite. Just a dab of purification oil and the bites are gone within minutes." ~ Jeanette

"During the late summer and early fall, I put Purification on my newborn daughter's feet every day to combat any germs my husband, a teacher and coach, might bring home. The baby stayed healthy, and as an added benefit, I noticed that neither she nor I had the usual mosquito bites that were possible year round in South Texas." ~ Laura

ITCHING (also see SKIN and FUNGAL INFECTIONS)

Rose and **Peppermint** – Place one drop of each into a ½ tsp. of salt and add to the bath water to make a Sitz bath.
Rose ointment – Apply to area.
Lavaderm Cooling Mist – Spray on area.
Clara Derm Spray – Spray on area.
Roman Chamomile - Apply topically and may be combined with Rose Ointment.

JAUNDICE

This occurs when abnormally high levels of the bile pigment, also known as bilirubin, in the blood stream can cause the yellow discoloration of the skin and whites of the eyes.

Di-Gize – Place one drop diluted with two drops almond, V-6 or olive oil applied to the bottom of the feet.

Place the baby near a window or go out for a walk in order to get 10 minutes of indirect sunlight daily. A mother's good diet, while pregnant and during frequent nursing, generally will abate newborn jaundice within a few days.

LABOR AND DELIVERY

Please note that as with many recommendations, mothers must take a 'wait and see' approach for the desired results. The amount of oil needed may vary from case to case depending on a mother's prior experiences. All of these oils can be diffused, directly inhaled or, two to four drops, added to bath water.

TO HALT EARLY LABOR:

Lavender – Apply a few drops on the belly to help calm and relax mom.

Peace & Calming – Apply one drop on the heart and solar plexus (chest), or diffuse.

Fennel – Apply five to seven drops to bottom of feet.

ENCOURAGE LABOR:

Jasmine – Apply as a perfume or inhale. Do not use internally.

DURING LABOR:

Labor Blend – Mix the following oils with ½ ounce of V-6 oil for use only after the labor starts. Massage two to four drops of the mixture inside the ankles, on little toes, little fingers, lower abdomen and back.

> **Helichrysum** (four drops)
> **Fennel** (four drops)
> **Peppermint** (two drops)
> **Ylang Ylang** (six drops)
> **Clary Sage** (three drops)

Frankincense – Dilute 1:1 and apply around vaginal opening.

Valor - Apply four to six drops on wrists, chest, back of neck and/or bottom of the feet. Wait five to 10 minutes before applying another oil. Also, diffuse one to two drops on chest, back of neck and base of spine during transitional labor/pushing.

Peace & Calming – Apply a drop to wrists, edge of ears, and/or bottom of feet.

Brain Power – Apply one to two drops on neck, throat, and temples and/or under nose. Also, one to two drops can be applied with a finger in the mouth on the insides of cheeks.

En-R-Gee – Apply along the spine and/or one to two drops to wrists, temples, back of neck, behind ears or feet.

Fennel and **Ylang Ylang** – Apply one to two drops of either or both on Vita Flex points on feet to advance labor.

Diffusing blend
>   **Lavender** (40 drops)
>   **Frankincense** (37 drops)
>   **Ylang Ylang** (21 drops)
>   **Roman Chamomile** (20 drops)

Diffuse in birthing room.

Washcloth blend – Place the following oils in a bowl of water, swish a washcloth in it and use it to cool mom's head and face.
>   **Jasmine** (10 drops)
>   **Roman Chamomile** (5 drops)
>   **Geranium** (5 drops)
>   **Lavender** (20 drops)

Afterbirth blend – Use the following oils with a carrier oil on the abdomen to help expel placenta and tone the uterus.
>   **Geranium** (10 drops)
>   **Lavender** (10 drops)
>   **Jasmine** (15 drops)

AFTER BIRTH, ANOINTING BABY

Clara Derm Spray – Parents spray on their hands and then anoint baby's head, face, around outside of eyes. Also, spray straight on baby's body, arms, legs and feet. Repeat for several days after birth as well.

Valor – Dilute 1:1 with V-6 oil and apply one to two drops on feet and spine.

Frankincense – Apply one or two drops on crown of head and anoint with prayer and thanksgiving.

Thieves – Diffuse in labor and delivery room to kill germs.

Peace & Calming – Apply one to two drops on bottom of mom's and baby's feet.

"Having used my YL oils, I felt so relaxed that it only took three swift pushes and our baby girl came only one hour and 10 minutes after arriving at the hospital. My precious husband called me 'Superwoman' because I got up out of the labor and delivery bed and walked to my private room on the other side of the hospital. That's how relaxed, yet revitalized I felt. The nurses were dumbfounded and in awe. The oils really kept me relaxed and focused!" ~ Karen

"We had our baby after only 1 hour and 33 min. labor. I arrived at the hospital door only eight minutes before she was here. Thank you for all of the advise and support through Gentle Babies during this pregnancy. It has helped a lot to know that I had alternatives to modern medicine when facing certain issues. Ningxia Red was invaluable throughout this pregnancy!" ~ Neisha

"I loved having the oils during my labor and delivery! Peace & Calming was my favorite and helped me relax. I was so excited to be able to anoint my baby with oils right after his birth. We sprayed Clara Derm with frankincense, myrrh, lavender and helichrysum on our hands to anoint his head and then sprayed directly all over his body and on the umbilical cord area. My baby's skin was so smooth and soft, and he smelled great! After the birth, I loved knowing that all of the oils I used would also kill any potential bacteria or viruses in the environment around us." ~ Sera

LACTATION

TO INCREASE:

Fennel – Swallow two drops of the oil in a teaspoon of honey every two hours. Follow with a glass of water.

Joy – Inhale to help calm and soothe as stress may have negative interference with lactation.

Prepare and enjoy the green smoothie on page 80.

TO DECREASE:

Clary Sage - Ingest two drops and apply neat to each breast two or three times per day.

Peppermint - Five drops orally several times per day. *Most herbal books will recommend avoiding peppermint during nursing as it may decrease milk supply; however, many mothers who have used peppermint report that it did not effect their lactation. See formula enhancers on page 52 if supplementation is needed.

"I have lost my milk around six or eight months with every child I have had. With my fourth I began losing it at five months. I read about using fennel and began putting a drop in my water bottle each day and rubbing it on my chest. I saw results within a few hours, and my milk supply is increasing. After Jack did not nurse for two days due to congestion my milk supply was low. I take one drop of fennel under the tongue and rub a drop or two across the chest, and my milk supply has visibly increased." ~ Beverly

"A lactation consultant determined the breastfeeding issues my daughter, Shula, had were because I was producing way too much milk, causing which my ejection force to be too strong. Pumping off the excess milk would be a temporary fix, as my brain still would be triggered to keep producing an overabundance of milk. My breasts had become painfully engorged with hard lumps in each of them, and my daughter fed for such short periods of time that there was no relief. I took two drops of Clary Sage orally, and rubbed two drops neat per breast twice the first day and three times the second day to decrease my milk supply. Also, I would hand-express milk for 20 to 30 seconds before each feeding to soften the areola and slow the ejection force without stimulating my brain to produce more milk. Lastly, I fed Shula every three hours, and stayed on the same breast for two to three feedings in a row. By the third day, my painful lumps and engorgement had disappeared, and my milk supply was in a much more manageable range." ~ Shannon

MASSAGE
See page 23 for detailed information about infant massage.
Peace & Calming, **Lavender**, **Di-Gize**, **Gentle Baby**, **Valor**, **R.C.** and **Joy** or **Relaxation Massage Oil**™ – Apply the oil of choice (others also acceptable depending on the desired results), diluted 1:1, on the baby.
Personalized massage oil blend
Start with a base of one ounce V-6 oil. Add to the base 10 drops of baby's favorite oil - the oil he or she responds to

best. To massage for a specific health concern, select an oil recommended in the Symptoms Guide under that specific topic. Label all blends for future use.

I recently worked with a two-month-old baby boy that the doctors wanted to operate on because the child was having lots of problems digesting his mothers milk. On all of my treatments for children, I first place one drop of Young Living oil and one drop of V-6 onto my hands before starting to treat the child. I massaged his stomach very lightly in a clockwise motion for several minutes with Di-Gize diluted with V-6 oil. I turned the child on his stomach and massaged his back (T12-L2) with the same motion using Gentle Baby and V-6 oil. I then started massaging the baby's body with Peace & Calming and V-6 oil. This child was fast asleep before I finished my treatment; he had been crying when his parents bought him into my office. This procedure took about 30 minutes. The next day the child's mother called me and told me that her baby had slept all night and had passed some ugly black mass in his bowel movement. This child had not slept all night since he was born and was always screaming in pain. The doctors had thought they had to do exploritory surgery in order to find out what was the main problem in the child's digestive system. Surgery averted. The parents now use these YL oils on all of their children in order to keep them healthy. ~ Margaret Nunez, L.M.T., M.T.I.

MORNING SICKNESS (also see NAUSEA & VOMITING)
Homemade herbal tea for morning sickness:
    1 teaspoon cloves
    1 teaspoon Turkey Rhubarb herb
    1 teaspoon cinnamon
    1 ounce fresh or dried spearmint
Simmer the first three herbs in one pint of water for five minutes. Pour this decoction over the spearmint in a glass jar and secure the lid. Let infuse until cool or twenty minutes, then strain. Take two tablespoons to ¼ cup every hour until nausea subsides. (Provided by Sandra Ellis, M.H.)

MOUTHWASH/ORAL HYGIENE

Thieves Mouthwash – Swish and swallow for fresh breath. If sensitivity to breath smell of labor support team, have them swish and swallow.

Peppermint and **Lemon oil** – Apply a drop of either to the tongue.

MUSCULAR PAIN

Aroma Siez – Apply as needed to sore muscle with a squirt of V-6 or other carrier oil.

Ortho Sport Massage Oil – Apply liberally for muscular and skeletal pain.

Marjoram – Apply directly on muscles or dilute with V-6 carrier oil.

Valor – Apply directly on sore areas and/or on bottom of feet and/or on spine.

Palo Santo – Apply directly on muscles or dilute with V-6.

Idaho Balsam Fir – Apply diluted or neat directly on sore area.

NAUSEA (see the NUTRITION GUIDE on page 77)

Di-Gize – Rub over the abdomen and put on drop on the finger to the inside of the cheeks.

Thieves – Ingest two to four drops in water. Apply a few drops to the feet.

Sandalwood – Rub one to two drops over abdomen.

PD 80/20 – Use as directed after consulting with a health care provider.

Peppermint – Apply on the tongue, one drop at a time. Also put a drop in hands and cup over mouth and nose, then inhale.

Lemon (or other Young Living citrus essential oil) – Mix five drops with a quart of pure water in a glass container and drink it all day long to purify the lymph system. Do not put the oil in a plastic container as it will react with petrochemical products.

NingXia Red – Drink one to two ounces a day in the morning.

Di-Gize – Rub one drop on inner cheeks of mouth and over stomach and inhale.

Melissa – Inhale and use in a foot bath.

Homemade herbal tea for morning sickness (see recipe on page 62)

Core Supplements, **JuvaPower®**, **MultiGreens™**, **Balance Complete**, **Mineral Essence** and **NingXia Red** – Use as directed to boost nutrition.

NUTRITION (see DIETARY REGIMEN DURING PREGNANCY and NUTRITION GUIDE on page 77)

℘ANIC (also see EMOTIONAL SUPPORT)

Peace & Calming – Apply on the body, chest and wrists or diffuse or use in a bath.

Lavender – Same application as above.

PERINEUM CARE (also see EPISIOTOMY PREVENTION)

ONE MONTH BEFORE DELIVERY:

Clary Sage (five drops) and **Rose** (two drops) – Mix with one ounce of wheat germ oil and apply to perineal area.

Myrrh – Dilute 1:10 with V-6 carrier oil and apply topically.

Clara Derm Spray – Spray each day or several times a day on the perineum, for the six weeks prior to delivery.

THREE WEEKS BEFORE DELIVERY:

Geranium (eight drops) and **Lavender** (five drops) – Mix with one ounce almond oil and rub on the perineum three times a day. This may help to soften the cervix and thins the membrane to get ready for delivery.

ONE WEEK BEFORE DELIVERY:

Geranium (eight drops), **Lavender** (five drops) and **Fennel** (five drops) – Mix with one ounce almond oil and apply on the perineum to further get it ready.

PERINEAL MASSAGE ONCE LABOR IS ESTABLISHED:

Myrrh – Dilute a few drops 1:10 and apply to perineum.

PERINEAL TEAR AND TRAUMA:

Clara Derm Spray – Apply several times, even hourly, daily.

Melrose – Dilute 1:10 and apply to perineum

Cypress (two drops) and **Lavender** (three drops) – Add oils to ½ tsp. of salt and mix into bath water to create a Sitz bath.

PINK EYE

Wash hands thoroughly when applying the following solutions: Express ½ ounce breast milk into a sterile cup cooled to room temperature. Use a sanitized dropper and place one to two drops in the affected eye.

Melrose and **Lavender** – Place one drop of each with one drop of olive oil onto a clean, sterile plate or a bowl with a lid. Use one finger to mix all together and immediately use the scant amount of oil on that finger to massage the outer bone of the eye socket, bridge of the nose, above the eye brow and the temple. There should be little to no oil residue on the skin after massaging. Be sure to use a small amount and avoid getting it into baby's eye. Nap time and night time are good times to use this formula. Cover the plate or bowl and reuse the formula twice per day; this is enough for several applications.

These essential oils, when used as directed, yield great results. Although a YL essential oil accidentally placed in the eye will not damage the eye, it may agitate it temporarily. If this occurs, put a few drops of V-6 oils to dilute it and the agitation should cease immediately. Do not use water.

PLACENTA PREVIA (see page 37)

POISON IVY

FOR EVERYONE:

ClaraDerm Spray – Spray on the affected area, repeat hourly until the condition is resolved.

FOR EVERYONE AGES TWO AND UP:

KidScents MightyZymes – Take tablets between meals (up to eight per day).

POSTPARTUM DEPRESSION (also see EMOTIONAL SUPPORT)

This may arrive with onset of lactation, one to four days after birth.

Thyromin™ – Two to three capsules at night to support thyroid gland function.

Jasmine – Add a few drops to ½ tsp. of salt and mix into bath water. **Ylang Ylang** or **Clary Sage** may be substituted for Jasmine.

Rose or **Joy** or **Idaho Balsam Fir** – Inhale and wear daily as a perfume.

Frankincense – Diffuse or apply anywhere on the body, direct or diluted 1:1.

Bergamot (two drops), **Ylang Ylang** (two drops) and **Clary Sage** (two drops) – Add to ½ teaspoon of salt and mix into bath water.

Feelings Kit – Use as directed or desired.

Progessence Plus Serum – Use as directed on bottle.

PRENATAL VITAMINS (see VITAMINS)

"Instead of taking over-the-counter prenatal vitamins, I chose with great confidence to take Master Formula Hers." ~ Karen

"My favorite prenatal vitamin regimen was Core Supplements, extra Omega Blue, and NingXia Red. I felt great!" ~ Sera

PUBIS DIASTIS

This is an abnormally wide gap between the two pubic bones and can be very painful.

Rose Ointment and Idaho Balsam Fir - Apply one or two drops of oil with the ointment and apply over the pubic area.

BLM - Two to four capsule daily as directed on the bottle for bone health support.

RESPIRATORY INFECTION (also see COUGHING and CONGESTION)

FOR BABY:

R.C. – Dilute 1:1 or neat to the baby's chest.

FOR MOTHER:
Peppermint, R.C., Thieves or **Frankincense** – Dilute 1:1 and apply to the feet several times each day. May also use Ravensara, Myrtle or Mryhh.

RESPIRATORY SYNCYTIAL VIRUS, known as RSV (also see COUGHING AND CONGESTION)
Raven, R.C., Peace & Calming – Dilute 1:1 and apply to chest area. Refer to onion and garlic poltice on page 42.

"When my son Caleb was just three months old, he came down with what seemed to be a very bad cold. He was very stuffy and miserable and couldn't sleep. The next day the pediatrician tested him, and Caleb was positive for RSV. Since my mother and husband had just been sick with bad respiratory infections that traveled to their chests, the doctor said the same would happen to Caleb. In addition, RSV makes some babies' oxygen levels drop so that they have to go to the emergency room, and I just could not let that happen. My friend, Sera, came over and brought her RSV blend of Thieves, Oregano, Raven and R.C. We applied it to Caleb's feet and diffused Thieves all day. He was still a little stuffy that night, but by the next day he was almost all clear and by the third day all signs of infection were gone! After that, I was hooked and have been using essential oils with my family ever since." ~ Wendy

RINGWORM
Melrose – Apply to area of concern.
Thieves Household Cleaner – Clean everything including bedding and clothing to prevent the spread.

ROSACEA (also see SKIN)
Frequently appearing on the face, eyelids, elbows and back, Rosacea, also known as adult acne, may take both internal cleansing and external essential oils to provide complete relief.
Lavender Hand & Body Lotion – Apply to the affected area two to three times each day until resolved.

SANITIZING

Thieves Household Cleaner may be diluted to various strengths for cleaning the whole house including babies room, toys, laundry and changing table. See House Cleaning on page 28.

SELF-ESTEEM (also see EMOTIONAL SUPPORT)
Believe – Apply anywhere, directly or diluted.
Valor – Apply on the soles of the feet or on the chest.

SELF-LOVE (also see EMOTIONAL SUPPORT)
For those days when mom may be feeling down:
Rose – Apply one drop on chest.
Joy and **Present Time** – Apply one drop of either or both as perfume on wrists and inhale.
Feelings Kit – Use as directed or desired.

SHINGLES
This virus of the herpes zoster family, the same as chicken pox, affects the nervous system. It may start with fatigue, fever and chills and involves extreme pain that can persist for months, even years. The skin will become sensitive to the touch and a rash or row of blisters will form. Anyone who has have ever had chicken pox may still harbor the herpes zoster virus and, when the body is under stress or the immune system is continually compromised, the virus may resurface as shingles.

Thieves and **Oregano** – Dilute 1:1 and apply topically to affected areas. Also ingest one or two drops of Thieves or Oregano in a 00 capsule.
Ravensara, Lavender and **Joy** – Apply to rash and also inhale.
Genesis Lotion™, Rose Ointment and **Cinnamint™ Lip Balm** – Apply multiple times each day or as needed.
NingXia Red - Drink a minimum of one ounce per day.
Shingles blend:
    Roman Chamomile (10 drops)
    Lavender (five drops)
    Bergamot (four drops)
    Geranium (two drops)

Raindrop Technique – Refer to the Essential Oils Desk Reference for instructions on this technique, which is very useful for all types of viral conditions.

SKIN

FOR BABY:

Rose – Dilute 1:30 with sweet almond oil and apply to skin.
Rose Ointment – Apply to dry spots or all over the body.
KidScents Lotion – Apply to entire body.
Animal Scents Ointment – Apply to the affected area.

FOR MOTHER:

Genesis Lotion™ – Apply to the entire body.
Mom's Skin Delight Blend – For itchy skin. Combine the following ingredients and apply the mixture as often as each day to wet skin after showering, especially on the growing belly. It may help soothe itching and could be beneficial for stretch marks too.

  2½ tablespoons of almond oil
  ½ tablespoon jojoba oil
  One Evening Primrose capsule (approximately 10 drops)
  One Vitamin E capsule (approximately 10 drops)
  Tangerine oil (four drops)
  Geranium (four drops)
  Lavender (four drops)
  Cypress (four drops)
  Lemon oil (three drops)

Drops of Gold facial ointment – Use the ingredients listed below to create this blend. Apply to the face, neck and arms for radiant and healthy looking skin. Recipe may be reduced for smaller quantities, but is best if bottled in 1/2 ounce bottles.

  Two ounces almond oil
  One ounce jojoba oil
  Two ounces Evening Primrose oil
  Vitamin E oil (40 drops)
  Patchouli (48 drops)
  Frankincense (40 drops)
  Geranium (24 drops)
  Palmarosa (16 drops)

Lavender (16 drops)
Rose (5 drops)

"During pregnancy I keep a bottle of Gentle Baby and Tender Tush in the shower. When I am done with my hot shower, I turn the water off and apply both to my belly – I did not have any 'extra' stretch marks this pregnancy. Wish I would have known this with my first three." ~ Beverly

"As my tummy began to get larger I applied a homemade salve night and day to keep it from feeling so dry and itchy. The salve, which is made with YL essential oils, started removing old stretch marks and kept new ones from appearing. I had the prettiest baby belly I had ever seen. I could have been in a magazine without touchups." ~ Karen

"All of my life I have dealt with psoriasis, which is a very complex issue encompassing diet, enzymes, candida, digestive health and even emotional health. The first thing I did to address the psoriasis, was to get rid of all of the toxins in my home – from my personal care products to household cleaners – and switch to the Young Living brand for toothpastes, soaps, shower gels, shampoos, conditioners and Thieves household cleaner. I also improved my diet, began drinking NingXia Red daily, cleansing and supplementing with Core Complete and a daily intake of essential oils. Three and a half years later, I found the psoriasis to ease up a bit ever so slightly around my body. In the Spring of 2009 I started using the new Lavender Hand and Body Lotion. After about a month or two of using this lotion, I realized the worst patch – on my left elbow – was totally gone, as were the patches on my hands and feet!" ~ Sera

SLEEPLESSNESS

Peace & Calming – Dilute 1:2 and apply on soles of feet at nap time or bedtime. Also may diffuse 20 to 30 minutes in the bedroom before bed.

Lavender – Same application as above and apply a few drops on the pillow or put bath water.

Valor – Apply on soles of feet before bedtime.

Tranquility Roll-On – Apply under the nose, back of the neck, soles of the feet and wrists. Also inhale.

SORE NIPPLES

Rose – Mix one or two drops in 20 milliliter of sweet almond oil or V-6 oil.

Rose Ointment – Apply topically as needed

Nursing Mom's Best Friend ointment – Use the ingredients below and follow the instructions on page 26 to create this ointment. Apply to dry, cracked nipples after nursing and wipe clean before nursing to avoid a bad taste in baby's mouth.

> **Geranium** (four drops)
> **St. Maries Lavender** (two drops)
> **Myrrh** (two drops)
> **Gentle Baby** (two drops)

SORE THROATS

FOR BABY:

Thieves and **oregano** – Apply neat on the bottoms of the feet three times per day.

Palo Santo or **Frankincense** – Apply one drop over the throat.

Thieves Wipes – Wipe neck and under ears.

FOR CHILD, ALL THE ABOVE PLUS:

NingXia Red – Freeze the one-ounce single packets frozen and serve as popsicles.

Thieves Spray – Spray once to the back of the throat. This may be a little hot at first, but will be soothing and fight infection. Repeat as needed.

Thieves Mouthwash – Gargle two to three times per day.

Thieves Soft Lozenges – Take as directed.

FOR MOM, ALL THE ABOVE PLUS:

Thieves Hard Lozenges – Take as directed.

Super C – Take several tablets spread throughout the day as desired.

NingXia Red – Drink slowly throughout the day.

STRETCH MARKS

For best results, rotate these oil/blend treatments.

PREVENTION:

Tender Tush – Apply topically a few times per day. It may be applied with Gentle Baby after bathing.

Lavender – Mix one or two drops with V-6 oil.

Gentle Baby – Mix one or two drops with V-6 oil or mix two to four drops with **Rose Ointment** all over abdomen.

Valor – Apply a few drops neat.

SOLUTION FOR OLD STRETCH MARKS:

Continue prevention protocol.

Gentle Baby and **Prenolone+Body Cream**™ – Apply topically each day after bathing.

TEETHING

FOR BABY:

Thieves – Dilute 1:5 and apply directly to affected area.

Exodus II™ – Apply one drop several times per day to relieve pain.

Clove - Dilute 1:5 with V-6 oil and massage the baby's gum and tooth area.

FOR CHILD:

PanAway and **Deep Relief** – Apply neat to the jaw over the area in pain. Help child to keep the oil out of his or her eyes; dilute the oil or have V-6 ready if this is a concern.

"As one of my daughter's molars came in it had a large pocket of fluid over it and the gum. She was in pain and had diarrhea. I applied a drop of Exodus II several times a day for pain relief. Within two days the pocket disappeared, and the tooth started to come through. Now she brings me the oils when she wants to taste or 'wear' them." ~ Laura

THRUSH (see also FUNGAL INFECTIONS)

Nursing mothers may experience an outbreak of candida in the form of an infection appearing in creamy white, slightly raised lesions stemming from the overuse of antibiotics. In addition, certain illnesses and stress can disturb the delicate balance of the body.

Life 5 Probiotic – One to two capsules daily to replenish lost intestinal flora.

Melrose – Place only a small amount on a clean finger and swab the baby's mouth. After five minutes, nurse to remove the taste. Mom: apply three to four drops over her lower abdomen.

NingXia Red – Nursing moms may drink one to three ounces daily. Dip a small amount on a clean finger and swab baby's mouth several times per day.

TIREDNESS (also see ENERGY)

Rosemary – Mix 10 drops in a teaspoon of Epsom salt and add to the bath water.

Orange oil (six drops) and **Geranium** (two drops) – Mix these oils with two tablespoons of V-6 oil for an invigorating massage oil blend to apply topically as needed.

NRG oil – smell, wear or use in massage.

TRAUMA (also see EMOTIONAL SUPPORT and PERINEUM TEAR)

Trauma Life – Dilute 1:30 with V-6 and apply to the mother and child after birth to combat physical and psycho-emotional trauma. Apply all over the body or directly on the entire spine and feet after birth.

UMBILICAL CORD

Myrrh – Dilute 1:10 with carrier oil and apply to the end of the umbilical cord for better healing.

Frankincense – Apply one to two drops per day directly on the umbilical cord stump until it falls off, generally in one week.

Geranium – Apply one to two drops for any bleeding around the umbilical cord/belly button. This may be diluted.

Umbilical cord ointment – Use the ingredients below and follow the instructions on page 26 to create this ointment. Apply topically until healed. To make a ¼ ounce portion, usually all that is needed, use:

    Lavender (one drop)
    Frankincense (one drop)
    Myrrh (one drop)

URINARY TRACT INFECTION (UTI)

Melrose – Apply neat over bladder area.

Lemongrass, Thieves and **Melrose** – One drop each orally in one ounce of NingXia Red or in a capsule swallowed with water, three times per day. Apply these same oils to the bottom of the feet twice daily.

Cranberry – Eat unsweetened, dried or fresh cranberries or drink four to six ounces unsweetened cranberry juice daily throughout the course of a day. Cranberry capsules also may be taken as directed. Because cranberries can be drying to the bladder and kidneys, do not take for prolonged periods. Blueberry juice is an alternative for those who do not like the tartness of cranberry juice.

K & B™ – Place 10 drops of this YL tincture into a small drinking glass. Boil one ounce of water and pour it into the glass with the tincture (this removes the alcohol base). Allow it to cool and then drink. Repeat this up to three times per day.

Juniper – Apply diluted 1:1 over bladder and kidneys.

UTERINE TONICS

Jasmine, Clary Sage, Frankincense, Ylang Ylang, Nutmeg and **Cistus** – Apply one or two drops of each or all topically over lower abdomen. Cistus may be especially good to rebuild and strengthen skin and tissue after caesarean sections weaken the uterus.

ITAMINS
FOR CHILD:

KidScents MightyVites – Take as directed.

NingXia Red – Drink at least one ounce per day for a powerhouse of nutrition, including B vitamins, potassium, calcium and minerals. The NingXia Red one-ounce single packets may be frozen and served as popsicles.

FOR MOTHER:

Core Supplements, Master Formula Hers™ and **True Source™** – Select one of these and take daily as directed.

VOMITING (also see NAUSEA and MORNING SICKNESS)

Nutrition is a must when dealing with vomiting as malnutrition and dehydration can cause additional problems. See the Nutrition Guide on page 77. Although the reason is not yet fully understood, lowered progesterone may play a role. Consult your health care provider before increasing progesterone. The following suggestions have been used to decrease and reduce the severity of vomiting and nausea.

Di-Gize – Rub over the abdomen and put on drop on the finger to the inside of the cheeks.

Thieves – Ingest two to four drops in water. Apply a few drops to the feet.

Sandalwood – Rub one to two drops over abdomen.

PD 80/20 - Use as directed after consulting with a health care provider.

Core Supplements, JuvaPower, MultiGreens, Balance Complete, Mineral Essence and **NingXia Red** - Use as directed to boost nutrition.

Progessence Plus Serum – Use as directed on bottle.

WATER BIRTH, DURING

Peace & Calming or **Lavender** – Mix 10 drops of either to bath water with ½ teaspoon of salt to relax.

WATER RETENTION (see EDEMA)

WHOOPING COUGH (also see COUGHING and RESPIRATORY INFECTION)

Roman Chamomile – Diffuse several drops about 15 to 20 minutes throughout the day. If a diffuser is not available, put three drops in hot water and place a safe distance from baby. This allows the baby to smell the vapors.

YEAST INFECTIONS (see also THRUSH)

An infection caused by strains of candida, especially candida albicans, that generally resides in the intestinal tract. This overgrowth can be present in the mucous membranes of the mouth and vagina.

FOR BABY (if the nursing mother has a yeast infection):

Melrose – Apply diluted 1:1 or neat to the lower abdomen.

FOR MOTHER:

Melrose – Apply diluted 1:1 or neat to the lower abdomen.

Life 5 Probiotic – One capsule in the evening after dinner. One in the morning if infection is widespread.

Inner Defense – One daily with meals, preferably four hours apart from the Life 5 Probiotic capsule. Limit intake of sugar and refined carbohydrates, which may feed the candida.

Nutrition Guide

"Who satisfies thy mouth with good things, so that thy youth is renewed like the eagle's." Psalm 103:5

Nutrition should take center stage in an expectant or nursing mother's life. It is critical to stay healthy and deliver the growing baby all the nutrition needed for him or her to be a healthy child. Making necessary changes to the family diet now will have long-term, positive habit-forming benefits. Here are some guidelines to follow while pregnant.

In general, opt for more homemade meals with an abundance of raw fruits and vegetables, whole grains, nuts, seeds, sprouts and quality protein. Some moms, especially as the pregnancy progresses, will find eating smaller meals more often is a better choice. Beware of spicy, greasy foods that are not nutrient dense and can be difficult to digest. Spicy foods also can upset the stomach of a nursing baby.

Most health professionals will agree that a daily multiple vitamin is in order. My choice is True Source, or the complete Core Supplements from Young Living (YL) Essential Oils; these are all-natural, food-based nutriceuticals. A great addition to mom's diet is a green drink to include extra vegetables for added nutrition. My suggestion is JuvaPower, a powder added to water, juice or mixed in with foods, sprinkled on vegetables and in salads.

Nursing is not the time to go on a diet to drop extra pounds gained while pregnant; nursing naturally helps the body shed those pounds. Moms who eat nutritiously while nursing are more likely to normalize their weight and have happy, healthy babies.

VEGETABLES

Consuming a large quantity of raw and lightly steamed vegetables gives the body loads of nutrition. Select a wide variety and make a big salad topped with legumes (beans) or lean protein part of the daily menu. Dark green leafy vegetables are good sources of calcium and iron. Include the enzyme blend Essentialzyme or the chewable KidScents MightyZymes if gas or bloating are an issue.

FRUITS

When consuming fruits, raw is best and in small amounts. The natural sugar from fruits can raise blood sugar levels for some individuals. A good afternoon snack may include a serving of fruit with nuts or nut butter (See recipe below under Nuts and Seeds). Fruit also make good desert options rather than high sugar cakes and cookies.

GRAINS

Avoid refined and over-processed foods, such as white flour, white sugar and boxed meals full of low-quality and unknown ingredients. Select whole grain breads and pastas for their higher nutritional value and low glycemic index. Grains comprise the largest carbohydrate category; some carbohydrates can raise blood sugar levels as much as or more than sugar. Elevated blood sugar level can lead to gestational diabetes. The doctor or midwife will check for this and make necessary recommendations.

NUTS AND SEEDS

Nuts and seeds are full of good fats that both mom and baby need. If digesting them is difficult, use them as nut butter on toast or bread. Available in many varieties, nuts also are a good source of protein and may be consumed raw or cooked/roasted. To make a truly delicious nut butter, put two cups of assorted nuts in a food processor or powerful blender and process until smooth and creamy. No additional salt or oils are required, and the taste is superb. Currently, there is much controversy over eating raw nuts and seeds. Although many believe eating them raw is more nutritious, an expectant mother should consult with her doctor or midwife.

PROTEIN

Turkey, chicken, lean beef, fish and eggs comprise the recommended animal protein. Legumes, nuts, grains and seeds provide non-animal protein. Buckwheat is the king of plant proteins and is easily added to baked goods and also found in cereals.

DAIRY

Plenty of calcium can be obtained from dark green leafy vegetables, but many moms feel the need to consume milk. Milk can be mucous forming and constipating, but if mom must have milk the best choice is organic raw milk from a trusted source. There also is much controversy over raw milk, and it is illegal to purchase it in some states.

FATS

Other than cold-pressed oils, such as olive, sunflower and flax, avoid consuming hydrogenated fats. Fried food is not beneficial to either mother or baby while pregnant or nursing.

FIBER

It is generally recommended that women eat 25 to 30 grams of fiber daily. Fiber can be found in whole grains, vegetables and fruits. A serving of whole grains at each meal will help mom achieve the recommend amounts. Fiber is important for proper bowel function. One serving of delicious Balance Complete contains 11 grams of fiber and is a great in-between meal snack or a breakfast meal on the go.

SUGARS

Always avoid foods rich in white, refined sugar including cakes, cookies, candy, pastries, some cereals and soda. Sugar has no nutritional value, does nothing for the body and can be potentially harmful. Moms who crave sweets can use honey, stevia and YL's Yacon Syrup in moderation.

WATER

Healthy water intake each day is estimated to be half the body weight in ounces. For pregnant moms, six more ounces should be added to avoid dehydration.

GREEN SMOOTHIE

Two tablespoons flaxseed Two
tablespoons chia seed Two
tablespoons sesame seed One
cup cold, clean water
½ cup ice
One medium peeled orange

½ avocado
One cup spinach
One cup or two to three kale
  leaves
One scoop of Pure Protein
  powder (optional)

In a blender, combine two tablespoons of flaxseeds, sesame seed
and chia seed and blend until it has the consistency of flour. Turn
of the off blender and scrape the sides of the blender to loosen the
seed flour. Add the rest of the ingredient and blend until creamy.
Add more water or fresh juice as desired.

• • • • •

Throughout this book various supplements and nutritional
suggestions are mentioned; the Resource Guide is on page 101.

• • • • •

FOR THE ENTIRE FAMILY

For a comprehensive guide to this subject, Growing Healthy
Homes offers a six-unit study co-authored by Debra Raybern titled
Nutrition 101: Choose Life! This family-friendly, Biblically-based
program overviews each system of the body and the foods that
hinder or nourish development. It includes detailed charts on
vitamins, minerals, protein, fiber, fats, fruits and vegetables and
healthy recipes in each chapter. It also is used as a curriculum to
teach children to love God's food. Order a book, CD, e-book or
combination set at GrowingHealthyHomes.com.

Birth Kits

Note: Essential oils and products associated with specific issues mentioned in the Symptoms Guide should be obtained in addition to the following recommendations and general birthing supplies.

BASIC BIRTH KIT

Essential 7 Kit — Includes Joy, Peace & Calming, Lavender, PanAway, Lemon oil and Purification.

Valor – Balances the body physically and emotionally and aids central nervous system relaxation and combats on-going aches and pains.

Gentle Baby – Helps comfort, soothe and reduce stress during pregnancy, prevents stretch marks and scars and aids prenatal bonding with baby and prepares perineum for labor.

Clary Sage – Supports labor, balancing of hormones and much more.

Fennel – Supports lactation, digestion and colic.

ClaraDerm Spray – Prepares perineum before birth and aids healing after birth.

EXPANDED BIRTH KIT

This includes the Basic Kit plus:

Trauma Life – Combats any trauma to the mom or baby, physically or emotionally, and balances the brain and nervous system. It is the most comprehensive oil in dealing with trauma and healing tissue.

Myrrh – Softens the perineum during labor, analgesic, anesthetic, heals umbilical cord ending and stretch marks, supports the immune system, spiritually uplifting, stimulates upper brain centers and master glands, similar to Frankincense, and more.

COMPREHENSIVE BIRTH KIT

This includes the Expanded Birth Kit plus:

Frankincense – Purifies, opens brain function, supports pituitary and pineal gland. It is one of the most holy oils for anointing the newborn. Aids in any type of wound healing, enhances immune function and more.

Rose – Because of its high frequency it is one of the greatest oils in affecting emotions and physical body. May help with healing trauma, stabilizing of moods especially during postpartum, relaxing, anti-scaring and deepens bonding with baby.

Dr. Mom's Wellness Chest

"But Jesus said, 'Suffer little children, and forbid them not, to come unto me; for of such is the kingdom of heaven.'" Matthew 19:14

These are the most commonly mentioned essential oils in this book. Be prepared with these oils at home and away.

Essential oils and blends included in Young Living's Start Living with Everyday Oils Kit include:
Lavender – For cuts and scrapes, burns, calming, blocked tear ducts, cradle cap and allergies.
Peppermint – For nausea, stomachaches, constipation, fever, headaches and other aches and pains.
Lemon oil – For coughs, immune support and pH balancing.
Frankincense – For colds, flu, pneumonia, bacterial and viral infections and the umbilical cord stump.
Thieves™ – For viral and bacterial infections; anti-fungal and anti-mold.
PanAway™ – For achy muscles and joints, headaches and arthritis.
Peace & Calming™– For relaxation and better sleep.
Valor™ – For backaches; anti-viral, anti-bacterial.
Purification™ – For insect bites, cuts and scrapes, coughs and bronchitis; anti-viral.

Additional Young Living Essential Oil Blends:
Melrose™ – For earaches; anti-viral, anti-bacterial and anti-fungal.
R.C.™ – For upper respiratory infections, bronchitis, asthma and congestion.
Raven™ – For upper respiratory infections and congestion.
Di-Gize™ – For stomachaches, stomach viruses, excess mucus and constipation.

Testimonies

"As arrows are in the hand of a mighty man, so are children of one's youth." Psalms 127:4

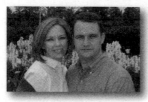

Katherine Grimes-Read C.N.M., R.N., M.S.N. and mother-to-be

I read a testimonial by someone who had used peppermint oil on her abdomen to turn a baby from breech (rear down) to vertex (head down). So I used it on two patients, and it worked on one and the other didn't turn. But the one that didn't turn even went to the hospital to have a version — where they manually turn the baby to vertex position — and it didn't work either. I will continue to use peppermint oil for first line treatment to turn breech babies.

Another mom, Sera, used essential oils throughout her pregnancy and delivered a 9 pound, 15 ounce baby a few days before her due date. She had about a two hour labor. Her placenta appeared to be healthy with no noticeable calcifications that are common with term or post-term placentas.

Karen Douglas, mother to four

All of my pregnancies were great, but my first with daily usage of essential oils was by far the best ...

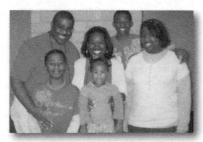

Before I became pregnant nutrition had become an important part of my life. I was drinking lots of pure water, eating a variety of fresh fruits and vegetables, and using Young Living Essential Oils (YL) and supplements. At the age of 40 I had my fourth child. Instead of using over-the-counter prenatal vitamins, I chose with great confidence to use YL Master Hers Vitamins, which have essential oils infused in them. During this pregnancy I used Valor all over my abdomen morning and night, Lavender on my feet, and Brain Power on my head. Also, I never left home without applying Peace & Calming to my wrists, the edges of my ears and the bottoms of my feet for an overall peaceful day. With prayer, my family and I used whatever oils we felt would assist me at that time and found them especially comforting, relaxing and revitalizing.

As my tummy began to get larger I applied a homemade salve night and day to keep it from feeling so dry and itchy. The salve, which is made with YL essential oils, started removing old stretch marks and kept new ones from appearing. I had the prettiest baby belly I had ever seen. I could have been in a magazine without touchups. I praise God that I walked in health the entire pregnancy.

On Sunday afternoon, I started having mild contractions. My husband Chris began rubbing Valor, Lavender, Brain Power and Peace & Calming on me. He repeated the process again at bedtime. I awoke at 1:30 a.m. Monday morning with strong contractions. Our oldest daughter, Brittany, age 12 at the time, knelt beside me and with her precious hand in mine began praying over me. Then she softly whispered in my ear that it was time to wake up daddy. At 2:45 a.m. with the oils in hand, we were off to the hospital. I was four centimeters dilated when I arrived at 3 a.m. From the time I arrived and was taken to my labor and delivery room, 45 minutes passed. It was time to push! There was no time to reapply the oils; the ones that were applied before bedtime would have to suffice.

Having used my YL oils I felt so relaxed that it only took three swift pushes and our baby girl, Faith Moriah Douglas, was born at 4:10 a.m., only one hour and 10 minutes after arriving at the hospital. Moments after her birth, Chris placed her on my chest, and we anointed her in the name of the Lord Jesus with the following oils diluted with equal parts of V-6 oil:
• Brain Power, which includes Frankincense oil in it that stimulates the limbic part of the brain and helps to overcome stress, was put on Faith's head.
• Valor, which also has Frankincense oil, was placed on her spine.

85

• Joy, which includes Rose oil that contains the highest frequency among essential oils, was placed over her heart.
• Peace & Calming, containing Orange and Ylang Ylang oils and increases relaxation, was placed on her feet.
• Lavender, a great relaxant, was used as a whole body message.

The aroma from the diffusing oils was so delightful that several nurses wanted to know what that beautiful smell was. After the birth, the doctor arrived around 4:15 a.m. The head nurse/midwife reported that I had a perfect delivery with no tearing, no IVs and no medications. I asked the doctor when I could go home and he said, "How about at 4:30?" However, I stayed for 24 hours only because Faith was required to stay. My precious husband called me 'Superwoman' because I got up out of the labor and delivery bed and walked to my private room on the other side of the hospital. That's how relaxed, yet revitalized I felt. The nurses were dumbfounded and in awe. The oils really kept me relaxed and focused!

I continued using the YL oils on myself and Faith and never suffered a bout of postpartum depression. I call this "my perfect home birth in a hospital." To this day, Faith still enjoys being rubbed with these stellar YL essential oils. To God be all the Glory! God's richest blessings on you and your precious baby.

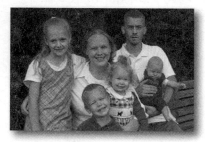

Beverly Boytim, mother to four
My two-year-old touched a hot generator muffler. We were a good way from our house and my husband put his hand under cold water while I ran to the house for Lavender. When I got back my son was in hysterics. I applied the lavender to his hand, and he calmed down considerably. We then took him to the house and continued with cold water and lavender. When the burning sensation had finally abated, I sprayed his hand with Lavaderm and applied a homemade burn paste; I then wrapped the hand in an ace bandage. Everyday I would let the burn get some air and the spray

again and apply the paste. Three days later the burn was healed and about 10 days later there was no sign of it.

I had a huge fear of pushing to the point that my midwife told me I held the birth of my third child about two hours just because I was afraid to push. I did not want this with my fourth, and I asked my naturopath what oils she thought would be good. I used Surrender and Release during the last three months, and I applied them to my wrist daily and smelled them. I did not have time to diffuse them during my labor though; it only lasted three hours with about five minutes of pushing.

Sera Johnson, mother to four

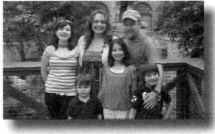

I am so blessed to have had my surprise oil baby, Ethan! This was my fourth pregnancy and was by far the best ever. Despite dealing with nausea the first trimester, — peppermint became my best friend— overall I felt better than ever. Because of the NingXia Red, Core Supplements, essential oils and a healthy diet, my energy stayed up, I didn't have any swelling, and my weight gain was less than my other pregnancies. The biggest difference was feeling so great overall. All of my labors and deliveries were short, but this one was the shortest and easiest — under two hours and I only pushed a few times. The most interesting thing was that my midwife commented that my placenta was one of the healthiest she had ever seen. Also, the nurse assistant noted that I had very rich milk.

Ethan was born with a condition called Torticollis where the muscles on the left side of his neck were too short and tight due to him being so big and being stuck in a certain position in utero. His head tilted to the left, and he had a bit of a droopy left eye. We didn't think much of it until he was about four months old and he still wouldn't hold his head totally straight up. A midwife knew exactly what it was and recommended I take him to a pediatric wellness chiropractor. I had never heard of this before, so I researched and found that if not corrected, it could cause physical developmental delays. With treatment, I learned it would take six months to a year to correct. So we started using the essential oils, particularly Valor, peppermint and PanAway along with the chiropractic and in two months, his head was totally straight and the muscles where perfect! Praise the Lord!

I really feel like a better mom now. Whenever anyone asks me if essential oils are okay for newborns and infants, I say, "Absolutely!" To God be the Glory! We are so blessed!

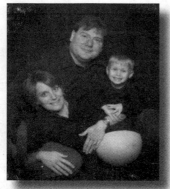

Wendy Stanziano, mother to two
Young Living Essential Oils and products have made such a difference in our lives and in the kind of mother I am becoming. Unfortunately, I didn't know much about the oils until after I had our first child, but since Caleb came home we've used lavender to help him sleep. After successfully relieving Caleb's RSV at three months of age, the oils have been an amazing tool for all the mild ailments infants have that can't be treated with over-the-counter medication. To this day, I use Thieves and R.C. for our whole family at the slightest sign of a cold and lavender for any burns or skin irritation. My husband used the Thyromin for an underactive thyroid and has normal hormone levels today. I am currently using Thyromin and Endoflex for my own hyperactive thyroid as an alternative to much more drastic treatments.

In addition to the oils, I believe that the NingXia Red has been an integral part of our health and wellness by building my whole family's immune systems.

A few days before we were going out of town to see family, I noticed red bumps/blisters on my son's feet. Because Caleb had slept terribly the night before, I immediately suspected hand-foot-

and-mouth disease. I checked his hands and mouth for blisters, but couldn't find any. He didn't have a fever or other symptoms. I chalked it up to teething.

By lunchtime, he had developed the blisters on his hands. I still didn't see any in his mouth, but I knew it had to be the virus especially when he wouldn't eat solids for dinner that night. Knowing we'd be seeing little cousins in just a few days, I began to apply Thieves on his feet and spine. I alternated with Mountain Savory and Purification.

Just an hour or so after applying the Purification, I tried to show the bumps to my mom, and I could only find two! I kept applying the Purification at every diaper change on Monday and continued as we traveled Tuesday. By Wednesday, the bumps we gone from his hands and only red spots remained on his feet! The cousins never got sick, and Caleb had a great time. He never seemed to have the fever, but the Purification really seemed to have shortened the duration of the virus!

Caleb, now three years old, takes Young Living's daily vitamin for children, KidScents MightyVites, along with NingXia Red. He's rarely at the doctor and avoided any type of antibiotic until this past winter. We also use the KidScents bath products on him and on our newest addition, Ava Rose. In fact, at just a few weeks old, Ava showed signs of a cold and congestion, which responded well to a little R.C. and Thieves in the diffuser. It's a great feeling to know that I have the power to use God's natural healing methods on my children! So many coughs, colds, tummy aches, and fevers have been alleviated with the various YL oils in the past three years.

Laura Hopkins, first-time mother
Young Living's therapeutic-grade essential oils are amazing because I can use them on my daughter, my husband, myself and even on our dog, without side effects. As I began to

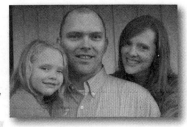

learn about them, I realized that God purposefully designed nature to provide these healing agents for us, His children. How loved and blessed we are! Unlike man's medicine, God created these oils to correct the root of a problem — infection, fungus, parasites — as well as the symptoms — fever, running nose, constipation.

My first experience was when my four-month-old, Audrey, developed a fever, I used peppermint diluted 50-50 with V-6 oil in her belly button. Almost immediately, it helped her have a bowel movement and reduced her fever, so I continued the regime every three hours. I also put Valor on her spine, and she was back to normal later that day.

Before eating, Audrey takes both her MightyZymes and her MightyVites three times a day. She also starts each day with at least one ounce of NingXia Red and loves to put on Orange, Purification and Peace & Calming. Between these products and oils and the Scriptures we confess about good health, she has never been to the doctor's office for anything other than a well-baby appointment. We have witnessed hundreds of testimonies in the past few years with family and friends of all ages. God is good all the time!

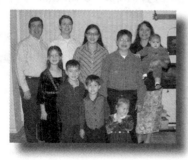

Jeanette Watje, mother to eight
I love to hear my two-year-old say, "Mommy oils, oils" and lie down with her feet up in the air! It also is hilarious seeing my teenagers crawl up the stairs so they don't waste any oil on their socks and can go to sleep with oils on their feet. None of my eight children have been seriously sick in over two years! We go places and are not in fear of getting sick, but if we do we are well within days instead of weeks like others that have the same sickness. We are praising God that we are feeling better and finding not only quick fixes, but preventive maintenance too. Instead of testimonies, I call these victories!

When someone is sick, it is a ritual for all my kids to line up with their socks at night and lie down so I can oil their feet, backs and sometimes chests depending on their illness. It is a blessing to see my children, who catch on quicker than I do, go to the oils first to solve health issues that occur. It is amazing to see God provide healing of so many things with the oils.

Kim Spendlove, mother to five

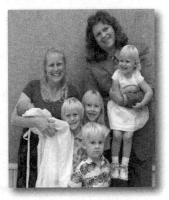

My fourth child was delivered via C-section, leaving me with an inverted "T" C-section scar; the surgery left me severely anemic and my recovery was very difficult. I did not known about YL essential oils at the time. After hearing the news we could never have another natural birth, my husband had a vasectomy. We immediately regretted it, and a year later the Lord made a reversal possible. We conceived our fifth child shortly after the reversal and once again were faced with the issue of our birthing options. Desperate to avoid another C-section we wanted to do everything we could to heal the wound. A year and a half had gone by, but we decided to try Cistus and Lavender applied over the womb area nightly to see what it would do.

I delivered our baby, a beautiful little girl in May 2008. We had a perfect natural VBAC without any complication. In fact, it was the easiest one so far. Even though we have no way of seeing my internal scar, the fading of my external one is substantial, and the pain and sensitivity I had are completely resolved. While I know oils were not the only factor, I am confident they played a key role in helping my womb to regenerate and strengthen making our VBAC possible.

I was in labor for 27 hours, and while it went very well, it was also extremely tiring. Several times when my energy was fading we rubbed Valor on my inner ankles. Within minutes I felt renewed, joyfully and any doubts that were trying to creep in faded away. As we neared transition my husband applied peppermint to my spine. I had a total of three transition contractions. The last one sent me from nine centimeters to 10, broke my water and sent our baby girl on her way into the world. Within a couple minutes and two pushes she was born. It was the fastest, easiest delivery I have ever had.

When my nursing newborn doesn't like something I have eaten I apply Peace & Calming over her tummy. Within about 10 minutes she relaxes and her spitting up stops completely. It usually doesn't return for the rest of the night.

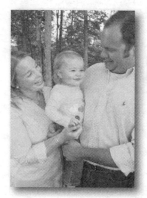

Jamie Hyatt, R.N., F.C.C.I., B.C.R.S., L.S.H., mother and grandmother

The minute my daughter, Emily, discovered she was pregnant the search began as to how to use Young Living Essential Oils during pregnancy, for labor and delivery and postpartum. Furthermore, she and I had a keen interest on how to use essential oils on a newborn infant. Within a very short period of time the book "Gentle Babies" appeared on my computer screen as if I had already placed an order. I purchased four copies, one for myself, Emily, her mother-in-law and an extra copy that I gave to a friend.

Emily's water broke at 9:15 p.m. Four hours later a Pitocin intravenous drip was started to facilitate uterine contractions. By 5 a.m. the next day only a few contractions had occurred. With permission from the attending physician Jasmine and Clary Sage were applied to the abdomen and on the inside of Emily's ankles to encourage contractions. This was repeated a second time about thirty minutes later.

Once labor began, a blend of Helichrysum, Fennel, Peppermint, Ylang Ylang and Clary Sage mixed in V-6 oil was applied to the abdomen, lower back, and on the insides of the ankles. Peace & Calming was used on the feet and around the edge of her ears.

Acupuncture was administered. Within a short period of time Emily was experiencing full labor. Because her cervix failed to dilate, the baby was delivered by C-section.

A healthy baby girl was born. Within minutes after her birth and held by her father, I was allowed the privilege of anointing my first grandchild, Isabelle, with a drop of Trauma Life on the crown of her head and Valor on her feet. Joy also was applied over her heart. Immediately following Emily's C-section a drop of Rose, Helichrysum, Idaho Balsam Fir and Believe were layered over and around the incision. Panaway was used for several days following surgery to eliminate pain. She used Lavender over the wound daily to assist with healing and prevent scaring.

Emily and her husband, Brad, continue to use various essential oils on Isabelle daily. Peace & Calming is their favorite oil. At twenty one months of age, Isabelle has been completely well, without any reported illnesses. Oiling Isabelle is part of her daily regime. In fact, she has her very own personal oil satchel which holds 16 of her favorite YL essential oils. Although the bottles are empty, she spends hours taking the lids off and smelling the essence of the fragrance — the perfect answer to a little girl who wants to have her oils on hand at all times.

Isabelle will become a big sister this year. Emily continues to use YL oils everyday and plans to incorporate them again in the labor and delivery process.

Becky Madding, R.N. BSN., mother to four

I am a white female whose weight has always been within the acceptable range for my height. I eat fairly healthy (never eat fried foods, rarely fast food, minimal sweets), I am active (keeping up with three toddlers and walking ¾ mile every night). No one in my family has ever had Type 1 diabetes, no one has ever had gestational diabetes, but I do have two aunts that have recently been diagnosed with Type 2 diabetes and both are on medications for it. With my pregnancies I have never gained more than 20 pounds and typically it was less than 15 pounds. Basically, I had zero risk factors for becoming a gestational diabetic.

When I failed my first glucose tolerance test with my first child my doctor was stunned. My numbers were high, but not so bad that medications or insulin were ever considered. I controlled my diet easily, and my glucose ranged usually from 80 to the 120's. Occasionally I would be high, but my glucose never went above 130's.

I managed to not have gestational diabetes with my second and third children. However, with my fourth I failed the tolerance test terribly. By this time the only risk factor beside my previous diagnosis was my age; I was 35 years old with the fourth versus 30 with my first. I failed so badly that my doctor wanted to put me on insulin immediately. The diabetic educators talked him into giving me a two-week, diet-controlled trial before going that route. When I initially started on the diet I was finding it impossible to keep my numbers down. This time my highs were in the 180's, and I was out of range at least once a day, but more often twice a day. I was so frustrated and had to almost starve myself to keep my sugars down, as best I could. I was absolutely fearful that I would have to go on insulin.

Then I got my NingXia Red. I started taking one ounce three times a day, following each meal. Within three to four days I noticed a dramatic difference. My sugars were in range (less than 120) almost all the time. I was usually high once or twice a week after starting NingXia Red, but when I was high it was only in the 130's not the 180's. After a week I noticed that I was able to eat larger portions and still maintain my sugars within range. That is awesome when you are pregnant and hungry almost all the time! I could not have done it without NingXia Red. Being diabetic while pregnant carries with it a lot of added risks both for mother and child, but if it can be diet controlled and controlled well the risks decrease markedly. I had a healthy, eight pound baby girl, full term with zero complications. Praise God!

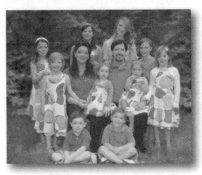

Christa Smith, mother to 11
As a young woman, I was very career-focused. The medical field was a natural choice for me because my father is an anesthesiologist and my mother is a registered nurse. After earning my degree in physiology, God directed me to nursing school, and my goal was to become a doctor. I worked for a year and a half on the OB floor of a teaching hospital and daily with physicians for nearly three years. Although I wanted children, I anticipated that I would have two and a nanny to focus on my career.

When we found out we were expecting our first child, the Lord changed my heart and I chose my family over my career. We had three beautiful daughters and I thought we were done. However, I conceived again and was overwhelmed by the idea of another child. Furthermore, at six weeks old my fourth daughter was diagnosed with the flu and RSV, both fatal to babies that young. During her intense illness and recovery, the Lord gave me new appreciation for life. I repented for my attitude and submitted everything, including my reproductive organs, to Him.

My first nine deliveries were induced due to preeclampsia or pregnancy-induced hypertension (PIH). The doctors used medications to control my high blood pressure, but usually it quit working at 32 weeks. I tried several medications, but I had to be induced because my body was so toxic – high ketones in my urine and high blood pressure that measured as high as 190/160. I spent most of my pregnancies on bed rest and was hospitalized at 31 weeks and given magnesium sulfate to keep my muscles from contracting and prevent pre-term labor. I had such horrible migraines, just sitting up would cause my blood pressure to rise.

Typically I was on the medications two months before and two months after delivering.

I was desperate. I tried juicing, nutrition supplements and just about anything anyone told me. I would swell and couldn't sleep. There was nothing that would alleviate this condition besides delivering the baby. During my ninth and tenth pregnancies, I used JuicePlus. I didn't have to go on medications until after the delivery, so I knew nutrition was helping. I had to be induced for both and continued to suffer from sinus issues, sciatic nerve pain and ligament pulls, which cause great pain in the upper leg and thighs.

Many well-meaning people were concerned for me and urged me to stop having children. However, I'd already submitted myself to the Lord. Early in my eleventh pregnancy, I attended an essential oils class taught by Karen Hopkins, a friend of Debra Raybern. I was interested in what the oils could do for my two-year-old who struggled with allergies that caused severe breathing problems. It was so severe that my daughter was on all fours coughing and trying to catch her breath. I made a rectal implant/enema with oils recommended for bronchitis. I watched her get up and start playing within 10 seconds. To God be the glory!

As a researcher, I wanted to know how and why the oils worked so quickly and effectively. I read Dr. David Stewart's book "The Chemistry of Essential Oils Made Simple: God's Love Manifest in Molecules." Dr. Stewart explained the oils could not be toxic and how they were safe and Scriptural. A couple of months later I attended a Raindrop Technique Intensive, giving and receiving Raindrops while pregnant. The class taught the chemistry of the oils, and I knew the oils were safe, non toxic, and were sent from the Creator. Surprisingly, I found relief from sciatica and also discovered that Lemongrass worked great when applied to ligament pulls.

I still was learning about the oils and had not really tried YL's nutritionals products. About 38 weeks along in my eleventh pregnancy, my midwife found I again had high ketones in my urine and learned I was hypoglycemic. Facing another induction and possible C-section, I called Karen. She helped me with a protocol of ingesting coriander, dill, peppermint, lavender and fennel oils and a nutrition plan with Power Meal, JuvaPower, Carbozyme, Life 5 Probiotic, Omega Blue and Pure Protein Complete.

I was shocked one week later with the results. Not only did the oils help, but I had no ketones in my urine and was no longer toxic. I realized that everything from PIH to my sinus issues were due to fungus – namely candida overgrowth. When I saw Karen a few weeks later, she said "You look like a different person!" Not only were the oils getting rid of the problem, but they were reversing the deteriorated condition of my body. At the age of 38, in the 39th week with my 11th child, I finally was having a normal pregnancy!

My eleventh delivery was an amazing, natural, vaginal birth. I used the oils recommended in Gentle Babies throughout labor, and we anointed our son with Frankincense as soon as he was born. I also put myrrh on his umbilical cord, and it fell off within 24 hours. Clearly we had an affect on the hospital staff because as we left the janitor asked if I had anything for her sinuses.

Our home hasn't been the same since we began using God's oils. I diffuse Cedarwood for congestion and sinus issues. I sometimes can't believe how quickly they work. We've gotten rid of warts with Frankincense, relieved congestion with Thieves, peppermint and Cedarwood, and dealt with sores with Lavender and Balsam Fir. When you have 11 children, you can really test the oils. I know Young Living has the best products because there is nothing at our house that they can't handle.

Evon McDonald, mother to 3 and grandmother to 8

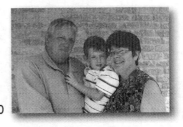

Our grandson Noah was given to us by the courts at the age of three months. Between two and three years of age, it was hard to watch our new son begin to exhibit signs of autism. Our first clues were what we thought was a lack of bonding with us. He did not want to be held, wanted to be alone and would not look at people when they tried to talk with him. As he neared three years of age, he became obsessive. The only way to get his attention was to touch him. He appeared to live in his own little world. He saw his regular doctor very, very often for sore throats, congestion, runny noses and earaches and seemed to be on antibiotics every few weeks. Our doctor saw the possibility of autism in his behavior and sent him to a specialist, who confirmed our fears after evaluating him.

A friend suggested I research essential oils instead of all the antibiotics he was taking. After research we realized that Young Living products were the best available. We began by putting two drops of Thieves on his feet every night; we used R.C. on his chest for congestion and peppermint in his navel for a temperature. We put Frankincense above his eyebrows and Brain Power on his temples every morning before he left for school. Between ages four and five, he only saw his doctor a handful of times. If I could not figure out what was wrong I would take him in for a diagnosis and then treat him with essential oils.

Noah is very intelligent. He memorizes anything he hears and can repeat extensive dialogues of movies. By the age of four, he could count to 150 by 2's, 5's and 10's, knew his phonic sounds and could spell over 40 words including all of the colors. However he would not hold a pencil to learn to write. He would talk to himself for hours while playing, but his vocabulary was memorized movie dialogues. He could not tell us if he was hungry or thirsty and was not potty trained at age five. He did not react to pain nor could he tell us where he hurt, but he angered easily.

In January 2009, I read about children with starving brains and learned how gluten binds to the receptors in the intestines and starves the brain by preventing the nutrients from being absorbed. After researching and going to the YL Convention, I realized YL had developed a product called MightyZymes that supplies a child's body with enzymes to breakdown many things, including gluten. I started giving Noah MightyZymes, but it was a hit and miss proposition. We did see improvement. He became more loving, wanted to be held and began to come and get us by the hand and take us somewhere to get something for him. In April 2009, he no longer wore a diaper during the day. He had very few accidents even at school and began to ask people their names.

In May 2009, I committed to give him three MightyZymes each day, every day. By the end of June, he burst out of his shell. His first sentence just blew me away: "Mommy, cook me some food." I knew that was not from a movie. He began talking in a conversational method and wanted us with him, to play, watch movies and read with him. During the first part of July we quit putting a night diaper on him. In January 2010, we had multiple family emergencies that distrupted our daily routine of applying oils and giving Noah MightyZymes. We began to notice regression in several areas and so did his teachers. This reinforced my belief that through YL's MightyZymes and essential oils, our Heavenly Father had released our child from many of the daily struggles of autism. I am recommitted to our previous habits of using YL products and am so blessed that we are all His children! (Matthew 6:33)

About the Author

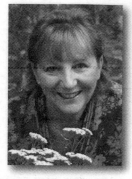 Debra Raybern shares her passion for health and wellness in the healing and restoring power of God's medicine; natural herbs, essential oils, right relationships and nutrition through semi- nars, lectures, books, magazine articles and personal consultations. Her vast knowledge, experience and Godly anointing has allowed her the privilege to help countless people with both minor and life threatening health problems by educating them in healthy nutrition practices, lifestyle, herbs and essential oils to cleanse and promote the body to heal itself.

Debra is certified in various holistic modalities, including naturopathy through the Herbal Healer Academy, a Master Herbalist Degree from The School of Natural Healing, as a Internationally Certified Aromatherapist by the Pacific Institute of Aromatherapy and as a Certified Nutritional Counselor with the American Association of Nutritional Counselors. She writes, lectures and teaches on the safe and effective use of herbs, herbal preparation methods and therapeutic-grade essential oils, as well as a variety of natural health topics. Debra's wellness articles have appeared in publications such as Countryside, Home School Digest, The Old Schoolhouse, The Link and An Encouraging Word. Her video, Whole Grain Cooking, and the recipe collection, From Our House To Your House, have helped many in preparing nutritious and delicious healthy meals. In 2009, she co-authored the ground-breaking book that serves as a family health program and curriculum *Nutrition 101: Choose Life!*

She is the founder of Sharing Great Health Inc., providing natural health and wellness solutions using traditional naturopathy and herbal remedies in conjunction with proper body specific nutrition since 1992. Her Web site is SharingGreatHealth.com.

Resource Guide

Essential Oils Desk Reference

The must have book for serious users of therapeutic-grade essential oils. It comes in three formats; large 500 page book; pocket size edition; or CD. The publisher, YL Wisdom, also carries a large selection of other natural health books, brochures and other resources. To order online visit ylwisdom.com or call 1-800-336-6308 to request a catalog and order by phone.

Nutrition 101: Choose Life!

Growing Healthy Homes LLC offers this ground-breaking, family-friendly, Biblically-based curriculum co-authored by Debra Raybern. All ages can learn from this three-in-one family nutrition and health program that presents the major body systems, how they function, their common health issues, the benefits of good food and the consequences of bad food. Packed with hands-on activities, science and art projects and nearly 80 family-friendly recipes, this program teaches and reinforces the why's of what we should eat. The 448-page book also includes a complete reference guide filled with nutrition facts, charts, practical tips and an exhaustive index and serves as a constant resource for improved health and abundant living. Available in a CD-ROM, book or combo package. Review an excerpt and order online at GrowingHealthyHomes.com.

Young Living Products

Young Living Essential Oils (YL) offers over 400 exceptional essential oils and essential oil enhanced products for health, home and happiness. Here are just the ones mentioned in this book.

Essential Oils

Australian blue
Balsam Fir (Idaho)
Bergamot
Cistus
Clary Sage
Cypress
Dill
Eucalyptus blue
Eucalyptus globulus
Eucalyptus radiata
Fennel
Frankincense
Geranium
German chamomile
Ginger
Helichrysum
Idaho balsam fir
Jasmine
Lavender
Lemon
Marjoram

Melissa
Myrrh
Myrtle
Nutmeg
Ocotea
Palmarosa
Palo Santo
Patchouli
Peppermint
Ravensara
Roman chamomile
Rose
Rosemary
Sandalwood
Spikenard
St. Marie's Lavender
Tangerine
Thyme Tsuga
Wintergreen
Ylang Ylang

Essential Oil Blends

3 Wise Men
Abundance
Aroma Life
Aroma Siez
Believe
Brain Power
Di-Gize

Endoflex
En-R-Gee
Exodus II
Forgiveness
Gentle Baby
Joy
Melrose

PanAway
Peace & Calming
Purification
Raven
R.C.
Stress Away

Surrender
Thieves
Tranquil
Trauma Life
Valor

Other Products

AlkaLime
Allerzyme
Animal Scents Ointment
Balance Complete
BLM
Cinnamint Lip Balm
ClaraDerm Spray
Comfortone
Core Essentials
Core Supplement
Detoxzyme
Essentialzyme
Genesis Lotion
Inner Defense
Juva Cleanse
JuvaPower
KidScents Bath Gel
KidScents Lotion
KidScents MightyVites
   Chewable Tablets
KidScents MightyZymes
   Chewable Tablets
KidScents Shampoo
KidScents Tender Tush
Lavaderm Cooling Mist

Lavender Hand & Body
   Lotion
Life 5 Probiotic
MultiGreens
NingXia Red
Omega Blue
OmegaGize
Ortho Sport Massage Oil
PD 80/20
Prenolone+Body Cream
Progessence Plus Serum
Pure Protein Complete
Relaxation Massage Oil
Rose Ointment
Thieves Foaming Hand
   Soap
Thieves Hand Sanitizer
Thieves Lozenges
Thieves Toothpaste
Thieves Mouthwash
Thyromin
True Source
V-6 Enhanced Vegetable
   Oil Complex

ORDER YOUNG LIVING PRODUCTS

1. Make a list of the products you would like to purchase.
2. Have a credit card or debit card or check handy.
3. Call Young Living at 1-800-371-2928 or go online to www.youngliving.com to place your order. You must have an Enroller and/or Sponsor number. This is the person who shared this book with you or who first introduced you to Young Living Essential Oils.

  • For online orders first select your country, then click on Sign Up. Follow the screen prompts by entering your personal information and the enroller/sponsor number.

  • You may choose to become a general customer and pay retail or become an independent distributor buying at wholesale and saving 24 percent. There are no monthly obligations for purchasing or recruiting and no yearly membership renewal as an independent distributor; this can simply be a wholesale account for your personal purchases. If you desire, you may initiate a home-based business, but it never required.

  • If you select the customer option, make your purchases and when the products arrive, enjoy!

  • If you select Independent Distributor, select your kit. (The author recommends the Everyday Oils Kit, as it contains many of the oils mentioned in this book.) Then, select Continue Shopping to order other products or complete the ordering process.

4. Be sure to write down your new Young Living account number, personal identification number and password for future order. Then, wait for your products to arrive and enjoy!

INDEX

True Source 74, 77
Tsuga 37

U

Umbilical cord 10, 37, 60, 73, 81, 83
Undiluted. *See* neat
Uterine tonics 74

V

V-6 enhanced vegetable oil complex 21
Valor 34, 35, 36, 51, 54, 58, 59, 61, 62, 63, 68, 71, 72, 81, 83, 84, 85, 88, 90
Vegetables 46, 77, 79
Viruses 28, 40, 54, 60, 83
Vitaflex 22
Vitamins 66, 74
  Core Supplements 64, 66, 74, 75
  KidScents MightyVites 35, 41, 74, 89
  Life 5 Probiotic 41, 73, 76
  Master Formula Hers 74
  Omega Blue 36, 39, 46
  True Source 74, 77
Vomiting 62, 75

W

Warts 97
Water 22, 46
Water birth 75
Water retention. *See* Edema
Weber State University 21
Weight 87
Wintergreen 56

Y

Yeast infections 75
YL. *See* Young Living Essential Oils
YlangYlang 58, 59, 66, 74

YLTG (Young Living Therapeutic-Grade) 14
Young Living Essential Oils 7, 14
Young Living Essential Oils (YL) aromatic farm land 18

To obtain additional copies of *Gentle Babies* and other books by Debra Raybern, please visit the publisher's website at GrowingHealthyHomes.com.

Nutrition 101: Choose Life!

Co-authored by Debra Raybern, this three-in-one family nutrition and health program for all ages presents the major body systems, how they function, their common health issues, the benefits of good food and the consequences of bad food. Biblically based and packed with hands-on activities, science and art projects and nearly 80 family-friendly recipes, this program teaches and reinforces the why's of what we should eat. The 448-page book includes a complete reference guide filled with nutrition facts, charts, practical tips and an exhaustive index and serves as a constant resource for improved health and abundant living. Available in an e-book, CD-ROM, book or combo package.